MIND THERAPIES
BODY THERAPIES

MIND THERAPIES BODY THERAPIES

A Consumer's Guide

George J. Feiss

Celestial Arts
Millbrae, California

For my parents and Susan
In gratitude, love, and respect

I would like to express my appreciation to Dr. Alan Moskowitz, Koen Kallop, Iris Samuel, and Tsering Pelden for their encouragement and support. Very special thanks to Andrew MacLeod for his fantastic artwork, his great sense of humor, and his unending encouragement and work in behalf of this book.

Celestial Arts
231 Adrian Road
Millbrae, California 94030

First Printing, August 1979

Made in the United States of America

Cover Design by Diane Hoyt-Goldsmith
Interior Illustrations by Andrew MacLeod

Library of Congress Cataloging in Publication Data

Feiss, George J.   1950-
    Mind therapies, body therapies.

    Includes index.
    1. Mind and body therapies.   I.   Title.
RC489.M53F44   615'.5   79-52334
ISBN 0-89087-247-3

1 2   3   4   5   6   7 — 85   84   83   82   81   80   79

Contents

Yoga, Meditation & the Martial Arts

Alternative Doctors

Selected Additional Topics

Preface

My intent in writing *Mind Therapies/Body Therapies* is to present in optimistically objective terms a factual resource book of the wide range of therapies available today. By optimistically objective I mean that while I have tried to view each discipline as objectively as possible, I have approached them all from a positive point of view in the belief that any one of them can be used by certain individuals as a tool for greater self-understanding. While I believe in the benefits of therapy, I also feel it is important to note that therapy, like anything else, can be abused or used as a crutch to feed one's problems or negative behavior patterns rather than to eliminate them. With this in mind, I still believe that therapy proves to be beneficial for the majority of the people participating in it—if for no other reason than it provides a supportive atmosphere in which to work on improving oneself. The purpose of this book is not to promote any one kind of therapy or therapy at all. It is simply to inform people about the great variety of techniques currently employed by therapists.

I have organized the book in six major sections, 1) Mind Therapies, 2) Body Therapies, 3) Mind/Body Therapies, 4) Yoga, Meditation and Martial Arts, 5) Alternative Doctors, and 6) Selected Additional Topics. I have done this as a matter of convenience for the reader based upon what I felt each technique focused upon. In actuality there are no hard and fast boundaries for any of these disciplines; all of them affect the whole (mind-body) organism to varying degrees.

In the past ten years the concept of therapy has been altered greatly for many people. Previously disdained by the *healthy* members of society, therapy was thought to be only for sick or weak people. The advent of the human potential movement (sensitivity training) brought a change not only in attitude but in the focus of many of the techniques themselves. Today more and more *healthy* people consider therapy to be an important part of their growth process.

Therapy is now being used not only as a means to straighten out one's problems or gain control over undesirable habits, but also as a valuable tool in the exciting process of self-discovery. Through therapy, people are acquiring increased insight into their relationships with themselves, other people and their environment.

This new approach to therapy has given rise to many new or *alternative* forms of therapy, the majority of which are covered in this book. The alternative therapies are so-called because they are alternatives to the old-line Freudian psychoanalytic school of psychotherapy. These new therapies are action oriented; they require that the client not only take a much more active role in the therapeutic process, but they are based on the premise that the client is totally responsible for his or her* situations and behavior. The new therapies are not a panacea. A person cannot go to therapy and expect to get fixed, happy or enlightened. Therapy requires a strong personal commitment on the part of the client and the desire to work diligently, especially when confronting difficult situations. In short, the success of a person's therapy depends upon how much effort he or she puts into it.

With the proliferation of new therapies (many of which are quite similar) it is oftentimes difficult to choose the best type of therapy to get involved in. No one discipline is right for everyone. Each technique represents a different path to the same potential place—greater self-understanding. The goal of *Mind Therapies/Body Therapies* is to enable the reader to get a feel for the options available, so that he or she will be better able to decide what if any type of therapy might be best for him or her. It is my hope that this increased awareness of the therapeutic opportunities available will encourage the reader to explore new avenues for utilizing more of his or her potential and thus lead to a happier, more fulfilled life.

George Feiss
Seattle, Washington
April, 1979

---

*A short note on the style of the book:

Due to the lack of a single pronoun that can be used to represent both men and women, I have chosen to alternate *he* and *she*, *him* and *her*, on a chapter-by-chapter basis throughout the book.

The asterisks in front of book titles in the additional reading sections indicate, in my opinion, the best books available on that particular subject.

mind
therapies

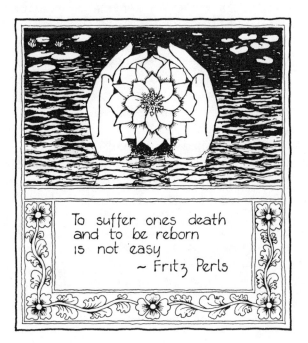

To suffer ones death
and to be reborn
is not easy
~ Fritz Perls

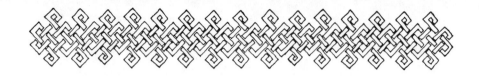

Gestalt Therapy

Gestalt therapy is one of the most utilized of the new psychotherapies. Developed in Europe, South Africa and the United States in the nineteen thirties and forties, Gestalt therapy has been an extremely influential force in the development of psychotherapy. The basic principles of Gestalt therapy stem mainly from the work of Dr. Frederick S. Perls, M.D., Ph.D. Dr. Perls, popularly known as Fritz, was born in Berlin in 1893. After completing his medical studies he became attracted to psychoanalysis and underwent training with a number of the well-known practitioners of the time, including Wilhelm Reich. He later came into contact with the ideas of Gestalt psychology and existentialism. During this period he was further influenced by the brutalities of World War I, and the rejection of his early work by his colleagues because he had dared to challenge the accepted concepts of the libido theory. Fleeing Nazi Germany for South Africa, Perls worked as an army psychiatrist, where he strove to develop more effective modes of treatment. There he established the South African Institute for Psychoanalysis in 1935. Upon coming to the United States, he created the New York Institute for Gestalt Therapy and the Cleveland Institute for Gestalt Therapy. Perls also wrote three widely acclaimed books: *Ego, Hunger and Aggression; Gestalt Therapy Verbatim;* and *In and Out the Garbage Pail,* an autobiography. During the latter years of his life, as he and his theories were becoming famous, Perls worked as a Gestalt therapist at the Esalen Institute in Big Sur, California. He died in Chicago in 1970.

Gestalt is a German word for which there is no exact English translation; roughly defined it means "the forming of an organized meaningful whole." Gestalt therapy deals with the individual as a whole, not as a summation of her parts, but as a coordination of them. Gestalt in this way is existential in its approach, for it deals strictly with the question of *being* rather than *having.* In Gestalt language a person does not *have* a heart, a liver and a brain etc., but she *is* a heart, a liver and a brain. The distinction between *being* and *having* is crucial in the understanding of Gestalt therapy, for by having something a duality is created—there is the owner and the thing possessed—while in being there is only one complete unit. This unit is made up of the individual and her environment. Perls stated that "one can't separate the organism and its environment. A plant taken out of its environment can't survive and neither can a human being. So one has to consider the part of the world in which he lives as part of himself." (3, p. 6)

The basic concept in Gestalt therapy is that of the "need fulfillment pattern in the individual as a process of Gestalt formation and destruction." (1, p. 1) Gestalt therapists believe that the phenomenal world is organized in accordance with the needs of the individual and that these needs both energize and organize one's behavior. An example of this is when a person is reading a book, the book is in the foreground of her attention. Suppose, however, that in the midst of reading she became thirsty. As her thirst grows the book recedes into the background, and the thirst becomes the dominant force in the foreground of her perception. Once she gets a glass of water and quenches this thirst, the need for water disappears. Upon returning to reading, the book regains its place in the foreground. The continual process of need fulfillment—as one need is met it disappears and another takes its place—is considered to be the dominating force behind one's behavior. This process, which Gestalt therapists believe to be a primary biological phenomenon, is known as the Gestalt formation. Perls believed that through the Gestalt formation process the organism or individual is able to regulate itself in the optimum manner. In a well-integrated person this process is going on constantly without interruption. "New needs are continually being formed; as they are satisfied they disappear to give rise to the next highest in the dominance hierarchy." (1, p. 4)

In an individual who is not well-integrated the Gestalt process is interrupted. The interference in the Gestalt formation, which is due to self-manipulation, results in the destruction of the organism's self-regulation. In Gestalt therapy the process of maturing is seen as the development from the environmental support to self-support. An individual who is not integrated will use her potential not for self-support, but to manipulate society by playing phony roles in order to gain environmental support. Self-manipulation takes place any time an individual does not accept who she is and tries to be different. Perls termed the two major ways of self-manipulation as the "topdog/underdog game." In the topdog game one is always telling oneself what she should or shouldn't do, how she should or shouldn't behave, etc. In the underdog game the person is defensive and feels that she has no power in her life. The underdog plays parts such as the victim, the baby, and other powerless roles. The result of this type of behavior is the "impasse," the point where the individual is stuck—she can't support herself and environmental support is not forthcoming. Perls uses an extreme case in point, the blue baby; it can't breathe for itself and it can't breathe through its mother any longer, so either it learns to support itself or it dies.

Perls believed that "every individual, every plant, every animal has only one inborn goal—to actualize itself as it is. A rose is a rose is a rose." (3, p. 33) Each time a person denies who she actually is, a part of her personality is lost. The result of an individual's not accepting and therefore trying to change who she is, is the destruction of her organismic self-regulation. The remedy for this situation lies in awareness, for as Perls said "with full awareness you become aware of this organismic self-regulation, you can let the organism take over without interfering, without interrupting; we can rely on the wisdom of the organism." (3, p. 17)

The purpose of Gestalt therapy is to help people regain the lost parts of their personalities so that they can become integrated. The method used by Gestalt therapists is different than that employed by most other schools of psychoanalysis, for they are concerned only with the present and not the past. While Freud postulated that people remain infantile due to past trauma, Gestalt therapists believe just the reverse—that people remain infantile because they are afraid to take responsibility for themselves in the *now*. "The two legs upon which Gestalt therapy walks are the *now* and the *how*. Now includes the balance of being here, experiencing, involvement, phenomenon, awareness. How covers everything that is structure, behavior, all that is actually going on—the ongoing process. All the rest is irrelevant, computing, apprehending and so on." (3, p. 47) In accordance with this philosophy, Gestalt therapists work directly and intensely with an individual's present feelings to bring about change. It is important to note that in Gestalt thereapy, change means—"becoming what one is, not trying to become what one is not." (1, p. xv)

Gestalt therapy is a step-by-step process of reowning one's lost parts. It can be done on a one-to-one basis or in a group. Most therapists and clients feel that the group sessions are the most beneficial, because an individual gets much more input from the group than would be possible from just a therapist. Dreamwork plays a large part in Gestalt therapy. Perls believed dreams to be the "royal road to integration." In Gestalt therapy the dreamer acts out each and every part in her dream, including inanimate objects such as desks, briefcases, whatever was in the dream—for the therapists believe that the dreamer is in fact everything in her dream. Another important technique is the continuum of awareness. This calls for an individual to be aware from second to second of what is happening to her. This might seem simple enough, but most people interrupt this awareness as soon as it becomes unpleasant. It is precisely these interruptions or times of unawareness that give rise to one's self-manipulation and alienation from herself.

In summary, Gestalt therapy is a very direct form of psychotherapy that is concerned only with how one is feeling in the now. The focus is on helping a person to regain the lost parts of her personality through the integration of attention and awareness of herself in the present. In doing this the individual will then be able to accept herself as she is. As the self-acceptance grows, she will be able to recover more and more of her disowned parts and thus will become increasingly more integrated. The more integrated one becomes the closer she moves to the Gestalt idea of health, "the appropriate balance of the coordination of all of what we are." (3, p. 6)

For more information contact:

There is an Institute for Gestalt
Therapy in most of the major cities
in the United States as well as in
many smaller cities and towns.

Additional reading:

1. *Fagan, Joen, and Shepherd, Irma. *What is Gestalt Therapy?* New York: Harper & Row, 1970.

---

*good initial choice for more information

2. Latner, Joel, Ph.D. *The Gestalt Therapy Book.* New York: Julian Press, 1973.
3. *Perls, Frederick S., M.D., Ph.D. *Gestalt Therapy Verbatim.* Moab, Utah: Real People Press, 1969.
4. Perls, Frederick S., M.D., Ph.D., Hefferline, Ralph, Ph.D., and Goodman, Paul, Ph.D. *Gestalt Therapy—Excitement and Growth in the Human Personality.* New York: Dell, 1951.
5. *Rosenblatt, Daniel, Ph.D. *Opening Doors—What Happens in Gestalt Therapy.* New York: Harper & Row, 1975.

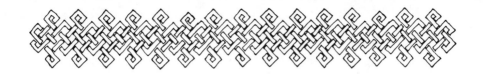

Transactional Analysis

Transactional Analysis, or TA as it is popularly known, was developed through the work of Dr. Eric Berne. Until his death in 1970, Dr. Berne was a practicing psychiatrist in Carmel, California, a Fellow of the American Psychiatric Association, as well as a diplomate of the American Board of Psychiatry and Neurology. A prolific writer, two of Dr. Berne's books, *Games People Play*, and *What Do You Say After You Say Hello?*, are widely read bestsellers. These easy to read and understand books have helped to spread the word about TA and establish it as one of the most popular of the new psychotherapies.

Transactional Analysis is a completely verbal form of psychotherapy that strives to give the participants increased intellectual insight into themselves and the various situations and problems they are working with. The first step in beginning TA is for the client and therapist to sit down together and draw up a mutually agreeable contract outlining what they will work on. This contract, aside from helping to form guidelines for the work in accordance with the client's needs, can be used as a marker by the client to determine whether or not he is getting what he came for. TA can be done on a one-to-one basis; however, the ideal format is group therapy. Since a large part of TA is structured around an individual's interactions (or in TA language, transactions) with other people, the group serves to create an atmosphere which demands that an individual not only become more aware of himself but also of how he relates to others. The group process forces an individual to look at his personality structure more closely, thus enabling a better determination of what needs to be changed.

The structure of TA theory is built upon the principle of helping one to gain better insight into four different kinds of analysis. These four are termed "*structural analysis*—the analysis of the individual's personality; *transactional analysis*—the analysis of what people do and say to one another; *game analysis*—the analysis of ulterior transactions leading to a payoff; and *script analysis*—the analysis of specific life dramas that people compulsively play out." (5, p. 16)

Structural analysis provides a way to analyze an individual's personality structure, i.e. thoughts, feelings and emotions based upon his ego states. Dr. Berne defined an ego state as "a consistent pattern of feeling and experience directly related to a corresponding consistent pattern of behavior." (3, p. 364) In effect, what this means is that a person, even when faced with a totally new situation, will not necessarily react to it in a manner that is warranted by the situation, if the present situation produces feelings and thoughts similar to those that were produced in a similar past experience. Every individual possesses three ego states—1) Parent 2) Adult and 3) Child. Each of the ego states is a separate and distinct source of behavior which exists in everyone at all times. The parent ego state contains the attitudes, feelings and behavior patterns which have been gained through interactions with other people, primarily one's parents. The adult ego state, which has nothing to do with an individual's chronological age, is the objective, information-compiling part of an individual's personality. The child ego state is where all the impulses and feelings that an individual had as a child are stored. When a person acts objectively in a situation, he is then acting from the adult ego state. The child ego state is most often stimulated in a situation where someone else acts like a parent or when a parent substitute is desired, a case in point being when one is ill. This ego state is associated with a wide range of behavior traits, some of which are—affectionate, playful, selfish, manipulative, and inquisitive. An individual acting from his parent ego state would act in a manner similar to the way he had observed his parents acting. Thus, an individual always has three different ego states to act from. One of the goals of TA is to help a person discover the patterns behind his actions so he will be able to act in the way he chooses, instead of acting compulsively in an ineffective manner from an ego state triggered by his old patterns. People continually act from all three states and it is proper and natural to do so, but it is important for an individual to be able to act in accordance with who he is *now* and not to have his actions in the present based upon his past experiences.

Transactional Analysis provides a method of viewing the interactions between people. Whenever one person sends a message (written, oral or through body language) to another person, he expects a response. In Transactional Analysis these interactions fall into one of three categories—"1) complementary transactions, 2) crossed transactions, and 3) ulterior transactions. A complementary transaction occurs when any message sent from a specific ego state gets the predicted response from a specific ego state in the other person." (5, p. 24) Dr. Berne termed a complementary reaction as one in which the response is "appropriate and expected and follows the natural order of a healthy human relationship." (2, p. 29) Complementary transactions can occur between any two ego states.

Crossed transactions are the reverse of complementary ones and refer to those instances when an unexpected response is made to the message that was given. In these circumstances an inappropriate ego state has been stimulated, and the messages have become crossed or missed completely.

"Ulterior transactions are the most complex type of transaction because they always involve more than two ego states. When an ulterior message is sent it is disguised under a socially acceptable transaction. An example of this is 'Won't you come up to see my paintings?' In this case the adult is verbalizing one thing while the child through the use of innuendo is sending a different message." (5, p. 29) Through TA a person is given the opportunity to see and understand how he sends and receives messages from other people. Once given the insight and understanding of why and how he relates to people, the individual is then able to make positive changes and improve his ability to communicate openly and honestly with others.

The analysis of psychological game playing is an important aspect of TA. *Games People Play,* one of Dr. Berne's bestsellers, was written on this topic. Berne defines a psychological game as "a recurring set of transactions, often repetitive, superficially rational with a concealed motivation." (5, p. 39) The problem with playing these games is that they prevent open, honest communication. These games by their very nature become repetitious, until one game feeds into another and no straight communication is possible. An example of this type of game playing is "Kiss Off." In this game of flirtation, which is quite popular, one individual leads another on until the second person has committed herself and then the game is ended by the first person. The player who had been doing the initial flirting received his pleasure from the other player's attention and pursuit. The constant repetition of this kind of game playing can result in the inability of an individual to have anything more than a superficial relationship with another person.

In the TA process the "ultimate goal is the analysis of the scripts, since they determine the destiny and identity of the individual." (5, p. 39) A script in TA terms is roughly defined as the life plan that an individual is compelled to play out. Scripts are formed in every child through the impressions made on the child by his early interactions with his parents. The first feelings that a child has of himself are believed to be the dominant motivating force throughout his life. In a very simplified example, a child that was loved, praised and made to feel like a good and worthy person is much more apt to lead a happy, constructive life than a child who wasn't shown much affection and grew up feeling that he was not worthy of it. These early feelings about oneself form the basis for one's life plan. The script then becomes, in effect, the stage from which all of the games and actions that take place in one's life are played out. Thus, by becoming more conscious of the games that one plays a person is able to become more aware of his scripts. As an individual's insight progresses it is not only possible to change the games, but also to alter his scripts for a happier and more productive life.

Transactional Analysis is a very viable method for getting to know oneself better. The intrinsically simple yet comprehensive structure of TA makes it one of the easiest forms of psychotherapy for an individual to apply to his daily life. By using the TA structure, an individual is provided with a practical point of reference from which he can realistically look at his feelings and behavior patterns and then decide what needs to be changed.

For more information contact:

There is a Transactional Analysis
Institute in most of the major cities
in the United States as well as in
many smaller cities and towns.

Additional reading:

1. *Berne, Eric, M.D. *What Do You Say After You Say Hello?* New York: Grove Press, 1972.
2. *Berne, Eric, M.D. *Games People Play.* New York: Grove Press, 1964.
3. Berne, Eric, M.D. *Principles of Group Treatment.* New York: Oxford University Press, 1966, p. 364.
4. Harris, Thomas. *I'm OK—You're OK.* New York: Harper & Row, 1969.
5. *James, Muriel, Ph.D., and Jongeward, Dorothy, Ph.D. *Born To Win.* Reading, MA: Addison—Wesley, 1971.

*good initial choice for more information

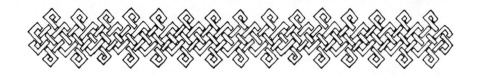

Re-evaluation Counseling

Re-evaluation Counseling is a unique method of psychotherapy in which the participants act as both clients and counselors. It was founded in 1952 by Harvey Jackins. Mr. Jackins worked as a labor organizer, poet and inventor before founding Personal Counselors Inc., the private organization which carries on the co-counseling, teaching and research behind Re-evaluation Counseling, or RC. Since 1970, RC has been growing rapidly and has now spread worldwide, with co-counselors represented in most of the large population centers of the United States.

The basis of the RC theory rests on the principle that people are inherently 1) happy, 2) full of life and energy, and 3) that they enjoy affection, open communication and the ability to cooperate with one another. The other aspects of human behavior which most people exhibit, especially the more negative qualities, are all attributed to reactions to things that have gone wrong, or "past hurts" in Re-evaluation Counseling language.

Jackins' belief is that humans are the only living beings that don't have preset patterns of response, that they can and do continuously create new responses to the situations around them. This is further pointed out by the fact that no two experiences or reactions to the experiences, no matter how similar, are identical. This ability to constantly see things as they are and respond in new ways to all new situations is what re-evaluation co-counselors consider to be the essence of humanness.

Jackins' concept is that positive information or experience is stored in the brain in a manner that will help the individual to act wisely in future situations, whereas negative experiences jam the mind in a way that causes it to become clogged or shut down. Thus, in times of distress, physical or emotional, people lose the flexible quality of their intelligence. Distress not only affects that part of the intelligence which is used to deal with it, but it also lowers one's overall capability to think flexibly and rationally. As people grow and continue to have negative experiences, a snowball effect is produced until finally there isn't much flexibility left in the individual's range of responses. Jackins sees the old phrases such as "I am losing my grip," and "I am not the person I used to be," as further reinforcement for his idea that the loss of a person's humanness is a process that takes place over time due to the repeated hurts one experiences during the course of a lifetime. The repercussions of a negative experience are not brought to a finish with the end of that experience. A detrimental side effect which accompanies all traumatic experiences is that it leaves the individual predisposed to be upset more easily the next time anything stimulates a similar negative response pattern. This, then, does not allow the individual to think or act rationally and clearly in the new situation, but throws her back into her old patterns which most probably were not then and will not be now the most effective ways to deal with the present experience. As this process is repeated continually, the inability to work freely with each new situation decreases until a person becomes rigid in her responses and has, in effect, lost her freedom. At this point the person has reached the chronic stage where she is acting as a compulsive recording of past behavior and feelings. Jackins believes in the philosophy of Rousseau that all people are inherently good and that they act in a bad manner due to the emotional injuries that they have received from their environment. Re-evaluation Counseling is a system designed to help people get back to this basic goodness through the process of discharging their old, trapped feelings. The objective of RC is to provide the space for people to feel safe enough to go through the discharge process and heal their emotional scars. It is the counselors' belief that the only real healing can come from within and that the actual process begins with the discharging of the old, repressed feelings. Everyone has been provided with the necessary "damage repair facilities" to successfully complete the healing process. These inherent qualities are "crying, trembling, laughing, anger discharge, yawning, and interested nonrepetitive talking." (1, p. 93) Unfortunately, most of the time an individual's healing process is cut short by others reacting to her in such familiar ways as, "Now, now, don't cry," or "Shut up," or other such interruptions. In this therapy the emphasis is placed on helping an individual through the discussion of her negative experience to discharge that experience and to fully use her "damage repair facilities."

RC is a unique form of psychotherapy in that there does not have to be, and in most cases there isn't, a professional involved. Co-counselors are individuals who have studied the Re-evaluation Counseling techniques and are themselves clients. Through this system of co-counseling, people are provided with a supportive atmosphere and a warm, attentive person who is interested in helping them go through the discharge process. In the next session, however, the roles may be reversed with the client now becoming the co-counselor, or both of them doing co-counseling with other people. Re-evaluation Counseling has been very effective in providing individuals with the ability to learn how to not only go through the healing process themselves, but to also help others become free of their rigid behavior patterns.

For more information contact:

Personal Counselors
719 Second Ave. N.
Seattle, WA 98109
(206) 284-0311

Additional reading:

1. Jackins, Harvey. *The Human Side of Human Beings.* Seattle: Rational Island Publishers, 1965.
2. Jackins, Harvey. *Fundamentals of Co-Counseling Manual.* Seattle: Rational Island Publishers, 1962.

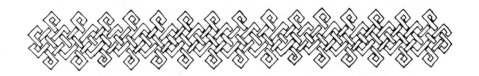

Rational Emotive Therapy

Rational Emotive Therapy (RET) is the method of psychotherapy developed by Albert Ellis. Dr. Ellis, a clinical psychologist from Columbia University, is well-known as both the founder of the Institute for Rational Living, and as a sex therapist. A prolific writer, Dr. Ellis has written many books and has received numerous awards including: Humanist of the Year, 1973; Distinguished Professional Psychology Award, 1975, from the American Psychology Association; and the Distinguished Sex Educator and Counselor Award in 1976.

RET is based on the premise that it is possible for a person to live a happy, constructive, fulfilled life, but only if he is capable of intelligently organizing and disciplining his thinking. Ellis believes that a person is largely in control of his own destiny, particularly his emotional destiny. This control over one's life is maintained by his basic values and beliefs. The way a person interprets or views the events that take place in his life and the actions chosen in response to these occurrences are seen to be the controlling forces behind an individual's emotional behavior. In RET theory the major problem lies in the fact that people don't act behaviorally or emotionally to the events that they experience. Rather, they cause their own reaction by the way they interpret the events, and most often the interpretation is influenced by an irrational belief. In short, oftentimes the events that occur in an individual's life do not upset him. The upsetting factor is the person's beliefs about those events.

Ellis created what he calls the ABC framework (although there are stages D and E) for getting at one's hidden beliefs. According to this theory, A represents the activating event, B stands for one's beliefs about the event, and C represents the emotional consequence. Using this method, it is possible to isolate an event, its consequences, and the reasoning behind the actions taken. Employed in this manner, the ABC format provides a person with a structure he can use to analyze his beliefs and determine whether or not they are realistic

15

and constructive or irrational and destructive. Ellis believes that there are a limited number of fundamental irrational beliefs. These can be fairly easily seen if one looks for 1) "musts" 2) "shoulds" and 3) unrealistic beliefs. Examples of these three guides to irrational belief patterns are: 1) "I *must* do well in order to win approval;" 2) "Others *should* treat me with respect;" and 3) "My living situation has to be arranged so that I get what I want quickly and easily, and so that I don't get what I don't want." (1, p. 33)

Once an individual has isolated the beliefs behind an action, part D comes into effect. D is the stage of debating, discriminating and defining. At this point a person goes through a great deal of internal questioning, examining each of the beliefs that pertain to the situation under question. As the process continues, one learns to discriminate between his rational and irrational needs, wants, desires and demands. At the conclusion of this stage, an individual's beliefs have been seriously studied and the irrational ones have been identified and weeded out so that they won't cause irrational behavior the next time around. The final stage (E) in the RET process is one of building a new, positive, rational belief system based on ideas that relate to the individual as he really is. This requires a reworking of thinking habits, behavioral habits, a restatement of preferences, and self-discipline in order to recognize one's true priorities. To accomplish this a person must be willing to work forcefully at modifying his dysfunctional conduct, because the old emotional patterns are not easily overcome.

RET is practiced in groups, couples and individual counseling. It is (in comparison to other techniques) a short-term, fast-results psychotherapeutic method that usually requires anywhere from one to thirty sessions with a therapist. The real work involved with RET, however, is the ongoing process of building one's new belief system. RET employs a variety of therapeutic modalities including role playing, assertion training, conditioning and counter-conditioning.

For more information contact:

Institute for Rational Emotive Therapy
45 East 65th St.
New York, NY 10021
(212) 535-0822

Additional reading:

1. *Ellis, Albert, & Grieger, Russel. *Handbook for Rational Emotive Therapy*. New York: Springer, 1977.
2. Ellis, Albert, & Harper, Robert. *A New Guide to Rational Living*. Englewood Cliffs, NJ: Prentice-Hall, 1975.
3. Ellis, Albert. *Reason and Emotion in Psychotherapy*. New York: Lyle Stuart, 1967.
4. Ellis, Albert. *Growth Through Reason*. New York: Institute for Rational Living, 1971.

---

*good initial choice for more information

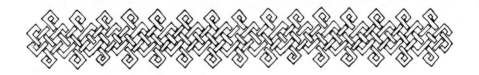

The Intensive Journal

The Intensive Journal is a method of psychological self-care developed by Ira Progoff. A former student of Carl Jung, Progoff is the director of the Institute for Research in Depth Psychology at Drew University and the founder of Dialogue House, a center for the teaching of his techniques.

Eugen Blueler, a Swiss psychiatrist, in the early part of the twentieth century first used the term "depth psychology." At that time he was using it in reference to Freud's theory of the unconscious. Progoff, the creator of the modern school of depth psychology, uses the word "depth" to stand for the dimension of wholeness in every person. To Progoff, depth psychology is a holistic approach, viewing an individual in her complete psychological state or in "wholeness in depth." Depth psychology is founded on the concept that everyone possesses the capacity for growth. According to the theory of depth psychology, everyone is also seen to have an inherent wisdom and direction in her life that is not always accessible to everyday consciousness. Depth psychology focuses on helping an individual understand her growth processes. As this becomes clear, a person is then able to get in touch with her inner wisdom and better understand the direction of her life. "The processes of growth are the processes by which what is potential in man progressively becomes more real, more actual, so that the meaning of man's life as a spiritual being in the natural world and in history is fulfilled in the individual's existence." (1, p. 373)

Progoff has devised a unique method, the Intensive Journal, which enables people to be their own depth psychologist. Created in 1966, the Intensive Journal is an instrument for a wide variety of techniques that aim at drawing a person's life towards wholeness. The Intensive Journal was designed so that an individual working alone with the basic text and paper and pen can contact her hidden capacities for growth, self-healing and self-direction. Through the basic text, *At a Journal Workshop,* a person begins to develop a dialogue with her inner self. Progoff writes (*Medical Self-Care* Magazine #4, Inverness, 1975, p. 4.) of "going down our own well until we reach the underground stream . . . We do not go down that well by analyzing or effort of will. Rather, we focus ourselves inward, relax the analytical, conscious mind and allow phrases, images and memories to arise on their own." As the images become clear they are recorded in the journal.

The Intensive Journal technique is quite different from the keeping of a diary or a journal of one's thoughts and feelings in that the Intensive Journal is structured and a diary is not. Through the structure of the Intensive Journal, an individual is able to expand the possibilities of the journal and get in touch with deeper feelings and images.

A fundamental belief in depth psychology is that every person is engaged in finding the way of life that is true to her nature. This search is aided through the regular and disciplined use of the Intensive Journal. A person using this method first learns how to reconnect with the continuity of her own life. With the continuity of one's life revealed, the inner guidance by which her life has been unfolding can be seen. At this point all of a person's past falls into place, illuminating her direction.

As stated earlier, all an individual needs to begin the Intensive Journal work is the text, paper, pen and at least two uninterrupted hours. The text, however, is not easy. It is highly recommended that a person interested in this approach to psychological self-care attend a Journal Workshop. During the Workshop, which lasts two days, one learns to bring her present situation into focus. In addition to this, an individual is taught how to use the journal techniques well enough so that they can easily be used privately once the Workshop has ended.

For more information on Intensive Journal Workshops
in your area contact:

Dialogue House
80 East 11th St.
New York, NY 10003
(800) 221-5844

Additional reading:

1. Matson, Katinka. *The Psychology Today Omni-book of Personal Development.* New York: William Morrow, 1977, p. 373.
2. *Progoff, Ira. *At a Journal Workshop.* New York: Dialogue House, 1975.
3. Progoff, Ira. *Depth Psychology and Modern Man: A New View of the Magnitude of Human Personality, Its Dimensions and Resources.* New York: Julian Press, 1959.
4. Progoff, Ira. *The Symbolic and the Real: A New Psychological Approach to the Fuller Experience of Personal Existence.* New York: McGraw-Hill, 1963.

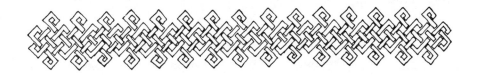

Reality Therapy

Reality Therapy is the unconventional approach to psychotherapy developed by William Glasser, M.D. Dr. Glasser, a psychiatrist in Los Angeles, is especially well-known for his work with juvenile delinquents. He was for a number of years a consultant of the Ventura School for Girls, the California Youth Authority and the Los Angeles Orthopaedic Hospital. Dr. Glasser has also been very active as an educator. He has worked closely with city and county administrators, counselors and teachers as well as directly with school children.

The cornerstone of Reality Therapy is the belief that *all* psychiatric problems are due to one basic inadequacy—the inability of the individual to fulfill his basic needs. Therefore, a person who is in a mental hospital claiming to be Jesus, a person with crippling migraine headaches, a person who is continually depressed, a burglar, and a person who suddenly goes berserk and starts shooting people all have the same problem—the inability to fulfill their needs. The severity of the symptom reflects directly the degree to which the individual is unable to meet his needs.

The two basic needs which must be met according to Reality Therapy are 1) the need to love and to be loved and 2) the need to feel worthwhile to oneself and to others. There is a key requirement to fulfilling these needs. An individual must be involved with at least one other person. The nature of the involvement is not of great importance (parent, friend, lover, spouse, therapist) as long as he has at least one person that he cares about and who returns these feelings. The other essential factor is that this individual must be in touch with reality and able to fulfill his own needs in a responsible manner. Without the key person or persons through whom one gains the strength and courage to cope with reality, an individual will not be able to fulfill the two requisites for good mental health.

The goal of Reality Therapy is to help people become able to fulfill their needs.

Reality Therapists view everyone, regardless of age, sex, race, and religion as being equal insofar as having these two basic needs which must be fulfilled. Everyone, however, does vary in his ability to meet these needs. Learning to fulfill one's needs is a continual life-long process which Glasser states "is best if started early, in infancy." (1, p. 11) This process is a continual one, for as an individual's situation in life changes he is required to learn how to fulfill his needs under different conditions and stresses.

According to the theory of Reality Therapy all people who are unable to fulfill their needs, no matter what behavior patterns they choose, have one characteristic in common—"they all deny the reality of the world around them." (1, p. 6) This denial might manifest itself in many different ways, such as a person who breaks the law—denying society's rules; a person with an ulcer who denies the fact that he is trying to do more than what he can reasonably cope with; or millions of people who drink or use drugs to block out the world they can't deal with. "Whether it is a partial denial, or the total blocking out of all reality by the chronic backward patient at a state mental hospital—the denial of some or all of reality is common to them all." (1, p. 6)

Responsibility is an extremely important concept in Reality Therapy. Dr. Glasser defines it as, "the ability to fulfill one's needs, and to do so in a way that does not deprive others of the ability to fulfill theirs." (1, p. 13) A responsible person is seen as one who does that which gives himself a feeling not only of self-worth, but of worth to others. Dr. Glasser wrote that "the teaching of responsibility is the most important task that people have." (1, p. 16) It is most often done through the loving discipline and example of one's parents, but if that has not been the case it is never too late to teach someone responsibility. For Reality Therapists, the teaching of responsibility is a central part of their work because they believe that at the core of a person's dilemma is his avoidance of the truth that, "one is responsible for his behavior." Dr. Glasser states that "People do not act irresponsibly because they are ill; they are ill because they act irresponsibly." (1, p. 32)

The goal of Reality Therapy is to help an individual (usually in a group setting) not only face and accept the real world, but also to fulfill his needs within the framework of it. A Reality Therapist helps to bring this transition about by first becoming involved with the client to the point where he can begin to face reality and see how his behavior is unrealistic. At this point the therapist is then able to confront the client with reality—asking him whether or not his behavior is responsible. Reality Therapy, like gestalt therapy, deals only with the present—making an individual accept responsibility for his life in the *now*. This is essential because one must be able to gain responsibility and fulfill his needs in the present. As Dr. Glasser states, "Why become involved with the irresponsible person he was? We want to become involved with the responsible person we know he can be." (1, p. 32) When a client admits that his behavior is irresponsible, the relearning phase of therapy begins. At this stage one of the major differences between Reality Therapy and the other schools of psychotherapy becomes apparent. Once the client has admitted that his behavior is unrealistic and irresponsible, the Reality Therapist helps teach him better ways to fulfill his needs. In more conventional forms of therapy, therapists don't believe trying to teach better behavior is a part of therapy. After a person has acquired more responsible behavior patterns it is only a matter of time until he is able to fulfill his needs.

In short, Reality Therapy is a process of intense personal involvement, in which one is required to face reality, reject irresponsible behavior and learn better patterns of behavior.

Additional reading:

1. Glasser, William, M.D. *Reality Therapy A New Approach To Psychiatry.* New York: Harper & Row, 1965.

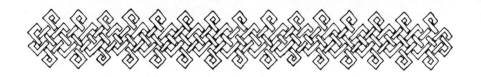

Psychodrama

"Psychodrama was born in Vienna, Austria on April Fools' Day, 1921 at 7:00 PM." (1, p. 1) At this precise time Dr. Jacob L. Moreno, the founder of psychodrama, was putting on his first psychodramatic play. Moreno, who grew up in a little town along the Danube River, was educated and began his career in Vienna during the era of Sigmund Freud and the birth of the psychoanalytic movement. Moreno, who had only one encounter with Dr.Freud, felt that his work in psychodrama came from diametrically opposite origins than that of psychoanalysis. He disdained the idea of meeting patients in the artificial setting of an office and instead chose to meet with people in the street. Furthermore, he stated that he didn't analyze dreams, but gave people the courage to dream again.

Moreno felt that Freud and the psychoanalytic movement had failed in two major respects. First, the rejection of religion, which he believed cost them the opportunity to study the saints and prophets whom he felt were the greatest psychotherapists before the advent of natural science. Their second mistake, he thought, lay in their indifference to the social movements (socialism, communism) of the time, which Moreno used to gain insight into group structure and group processes. This study of the group led him to become the first person to use group therapy. "Historically, psychodrama represents the chief turning point away from the treatment of the individual in isolation, to the treatment of the individual in groups, from the treatment of the individual by verbal methods to the treatment by action methods." (1, p. 10)

Psychodrama is the form of psychotherapy that employs acting to help the patient solve her problems. Under the guidance of a director (a therapist) the client acts out situations and relationships that are disturbing to her. Other members of the group are often used to play the roles of the different people involved in the client's particular problem (i.e. mother, father, husband). "The client is encouraged to walk around the stage, talk and act out a series of episodes that are spontaneously produced—a direct expression of various life situations related to his difficulties. The many techniques of the method elicit responses that reveal personality traits and particular modes of action." (2, p. 11)

Psychodrama is a very dramatic form of group psychotherapy. The action of acting out one's problems in a group setting enables a person to not only gain greater insight into her problems, but also provides a supportive atmosphere for an individual to experience a "catharsis," or deep release of tension. "The catharsis is brought on by the individual acting and reliving events that he previously had not been able to understand." (2, p. 3) As a person's awareness concerning her problems increases, the tension built up due to these problems is released.

Psychodrama is practiced by both psychologists and psychiatrists. For more information contact:

American Society of Group Psychotherapy
and Psychodrama
39 East 20th St.
New York, NY 10003
(212) 260-3860

1. Moreno, Jacob L. *Psychodrama.* New York: Beacon House, 1946, p. 1.
2. Starr, Adaline. *Psychodrama Rehearsal For Living.* Chicago: Nelson Hall, 1978, p. 3.

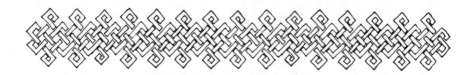

Psychosynthesis

Psychosynthesis is an eclectic, comprehensive form of psychotherapy based on the discovery and expansion of the self. Roberto Assagioli, an Italian psychiatrist and colleague of Freud and Jung, founded Psychosynthesis in 1911. Assagioli, one of the pioneers of psychotherapy in Italy, felt that Freudian psychoanalysis did not place enough importance on the "higher" attributes of people. As a student of both Eastern and Western philosophical and spiritual traditions, Assagioli believed that in order to develop a truly inclusive conception of the human being, it was of the utmost importance to study the transpersonal dimension ("a higher center of being which transcends even the duality of individuality and universality") of a person's experience as well as the development of his personality. In 1926 the Institute of Psychosynthesis was established in Rome for the purposes of further research, development and teaching of the techniques used by the practitioners of Psychosynthesis.

The guiding concepts of Psychosynthesis are that an individual is in a constant state of growth; that one actualizes his hidden potential through the ability to make decisions and choices as well as through the importance that he assigns to different value systems (ethical, religious and aesthetic).

According to the theory of Psychosynthesis, every individual is made up of seven parts: "1) *The Lower Unconscious* which contains the fundamental drives, primitive urges and the elementary physiological activities which direct the life of the body . . . 2) *The Middle Unconscious* is formed of psychological elements similar to those of one's waking consciousness . . . 3) *The Higher Unconscious* or *Superconscious* is the source of higher feelings such as love, genius and states of contemplation . . . 4) *The Field of Consciousness* represents that part of one's personality of which he is directly aware— thoughts, feelings and desires . . . 5) *The Conscious Self* or *I* is the "Self" or the point of pure self-awareness . . . 6) *The Higher Self* is a true self that exists beyond the body . . . And, 7) *The Collective Unconscious* encompasses all of the first six parts of one's being. . ." (1, p. 17)

The aim of Psychosynthesis is a thorough integration of these seven states of consciousness. This is achieved through a four-stage process. The first step is for an individual to learn about the various elements involved in the makeup of his personality. This requires more than a cursory study of his habits and traits. The depths of one's unconscious, where the images of childhood, fear and conflict are stored, must be explored. This procedure can be done alone or with the help of a therapist. In the second stage one learns to control the elements of his personality through the process of disidentification. This method is based upon the psychological principle that a person becomes dominated by everything with which the self becomes identified. "Every time we identify ourselves with a weakness, a fault, or fear or any personal emotion or drive, we limit and paralyze ourselves. Every time we admit, 'I am discouraged,' or 'I am irritated,' we become more and more dominated by depression or anger. We have accepted those limitations; we have ourselves put on our chains. If, instead, in the same situation we say, 'A wave of discouragement is *trying* to submerge me,' or 'An impulse of anger is attempting to overpower me,' the situation is very different. Then there are two forces confronting each other—on one side, our vigilant self and, on the other, the discouragement or the anger. And the vigilant self does not submit to that invasion; it can objectively and critically survey those impulses of discouragement or anger; it can look for their origin, foresee their deleterious effects, and realize their unfoundedness." (1, p. 22) In order to separate oneself from these images, the methods of objectification, critical analysis and discrimination are used. Maintaining a psychological distance between the self and the destructive images enables a person to redirect the energy that is usually spent in keeping the negative images alive into a more creative channel. The third stage of integration involves the expansion of one's personal consciousness into the real self. Through this a person discovers his psychological center. In the fourth stage, the stage of Psychosynthesis, the newly discovered psychological center is reinforced with a unified, coherent and organized personality.

Psychosynthesis can be done individually or in groups. Practitioners use a wide range of methods and are not limited to those developed by or through Psychosynthesis. Among the techniques regularly employed are dream analysis, psychodrama, guided imagery, use of diaries and Gestalt therapy.

For more information contact:

Psychosynthesis Institute
3352 Sacramento St.
San Francisco, CA 94118
(415) 922-9182

Canadian Institute of
Psychosynthesis
3496 Marlowe Ave.
Montreal, Quebec
H4A 3L7 Canada
(514) 488-4494

Additional reading:

1. Assagioli, Roberto. *Psychosynthesis*. New York: Hobbs, Dorman & Co., 1965

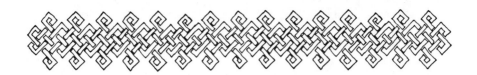

Fischer–Hoffman

The Fischer–Hoffman Process is a unique form of psychotherapy in just about every respect, from the way it was developed to its actual techniques. One night in 1967 the psychic Bob Hoffman contacted the spirit of his old friend, Dr. Siegfried Fischer. In the six months since his death, Dr. Fischer had put together a new form of "emotional healing" which he proceeded to teach Hoffman for the next five hours. This psychic transmission forms the basis of the Fischer–Hoffman Process. The theory and procedures of the process have been continually refined and expanded upon over the last ten years under the guidance of Dr. Fischer.

Practitioners of the Fischer–Hoffman Process view an individual as a quadrinity. Everyone is not only a physical being but also a three-part nonphysical entity. The body is the physical aspect of the self. The nonphysical components are: 1) the emotional self, the child within each person that stopped growing emotionally at the time of puberty; 2) the individual's intellectual self at her present age; and 3) the timeless spiritual self. The Fischer–Hoffman Process is designed to facilitate an individual's re-education of her emotional child, to enable her to finally drop her childish "negative love" patterns. Through this process the emotional child grows up to the individual's present chronological and intellectual age, retaining its positive childlike qualities (spontaneity, curiosity, humor) while ridding itself of the negative childish ones (needy, demanding, manipulative). As the emotional child matures, the quadrinity (body, emotions, intellect, and spirit) becomes fully integrated, ending not only the split between one's different parts but also the inner turmoil and confusion that results when a person does not function as an emotionally whole being.

The Fischer–Hoffman Process rests firmly on the belief that the negative feelings one encountered so frequently in one's life are not inevitable, but are learned responses to certain situations and stimuli that can be unlearned through re-education. The emphasis of the Fis-cher–Hoffman Process, as in many therapies, is placed on helping a person to really love herself. In order to accomplish this the process employs a unique approach to an old problem. The focus of this therapy is on an individual's relationship with her parents in the be-lief that this crucial relationship provides the major training ground for learning how to love oneself and others. The technique is de-signed to help a person get a "loving divorce from her mother and father (whether they are still living or not)." The concept underlying this approach is that the way a child is loved by her parents is the model the child will have for not only loving herself but others as well. "All emotional problems are thought to be the result of nega-tive love. When a person adopts the negative traits, moods and ad-monitions of her parents in the hope of getting the unconditional love and acceptance which are one's greatest needs as a child, that is the negative love syndrome. Rebelling against Mother and Father, which always leads to internal conflict (because then you won't get their love), is only another aspect of the same thing." (2)

The Fischer–Hoffman Process is also unique in that the majority of the work which takes place during the time one is in therapy is not verbal or action oriented, but written. The process consists of one "non-encounter group session" a week for thirteen weeks. During each session the therapist speaks while the clients take pages and pages of notes. At the end of each group meeting an assignment is given which is supposed to be written out and sent in during the week. An example of one such assignment is a "25-page negative emotional autobiography of one's relationship with her mother." (2)

Upon returning to the next session a highly detailed tape cassette is given to each client containing the therapist's insights on a line-by-line basis of what she had written during the week. As the therapy progresses a person experiences the following stages of psychological and emotional development. "First the client prosecutes both Mother and Father for the crime that they committed by bringing her up to be unloving and neurotic. After all the anger is released the client then goes through a period of defending her parents. The next stage brings to an end the war between one's intellect and emotional child. By the end of the thirteenth session the individual has become an in-tegrated whole being through the joining of the *matured* emotional self to her intellectual and spiritual self." (2)

Once this has been accomplished the client is not only able to express both love and compassion for her parents, but more importantly is genuinely capable of loving herself.

For more information contact:

> Hoffman Quadrinity Center
> 1005 Sansome St.
> San Francisco, CA 94111
> (415) 397-0466

Additional reading:

1. Hoffman, Bob. *Getting Divorced from Mother and Dad.* New York: E.P. Dutton, 1976.
2. Pastor, Marion. The Fischer–Hoffman Process— An Alternative to Therapy. San Francisco: Hoffman Quadrinity Center, 1975.

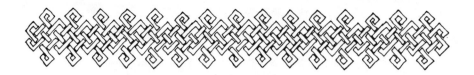

Biofeedback

Biofeedback is a method that employs advanced technology as a tool for self-discovery and greater conscious control over one's involuntary nervous system. The body contains two nervous systems, the functions of which are quite different. The central or somatic nervous system is comprised of the brain, the twelve pairs of nerves that regulate its impulses, and the thirty-one pairs of nerves that run throughout the body from their housing inside the spinal column. The central nervous system controls the entire skeleton, the muscles and all of the movements made by the limbs. The autonomic (involuntary) nervous system is located along the spinal column and is in charge of the functioning of the body inside the skeletal frame. It controls the operation of the internal organs, the glands, the respiratory and the circulatory systems. The idea that an individual is capable of controlling the functioning of his autonomic (involuntary) nervous system has until recently been espoused only by mystics and yogis. The advent of Biofeedback, however, has changed the thinking of many people by giving Western scientists proof that at the very least some of the functions of the autonomic nervous system are subject to a limited amount of conscious control.

In 1929 Hans Berger, a German doctor, brought the concept of Biofeedback to the attention of the scientific world. Dr. Berger published a paper in which he discussed his work of monitoring the electroencephalograms (EEG—a measurement of the brain's electrical signals) of human subjects by attaching electrodes from his galvanometer to their scalps. Dr. Berger noticed that not only did the brain waves vary in frequency and amplitude but the changes seemed to correspond to changes in consciousness. This was the discovery of the alpha and beta brain waves. Progress in the area of brain wave feedback was slow until the 1950s when Barbara Brown, Joe Kayima and Elmer Green discovered that Biofeedback (the use of information from psychological measuring instruments) could be used effectively in training people to gain voluntary control over their involuntary processes. A Biofeedback machine is used as an extension of the five senses. It monitors one's inner states such as the structural activity of the heart, brain, blood circulation and respiration, and then feeds back the information in much the same manner as any of the other senses. "In effect, it provides a new or sixth sense that causes awareness of mind/body processes that were previously unconscious. By paying attention to this new information and being willing to make the effort to learn, one can gain control of the mind/body process being measured. Thus, Biofeedback instruments are simply measuring tools that can be adapted as teaching machines." (1, p. 203)

Brain waves are categorized in four distinct groups according to their frequencies, which are measured in Hertz (Hz—cycles per second). These different rhythms are thought to be the result of the electrical impulses given off by the brain as it relays various types of information to different parts of the body. The beta waves, which have a frequency of more than 13Hz, are commonly associated with the active working or playing state. As an individual relaxes, the beta wave pattern gives way to alpha waves which range in frequency from 8–13Hz. The theta waves, which have a range of 4–8Hz, come into play in the stage where a person becomes drowsy and passes into light sleep. "As a general rule of thumb, it can be said that beta waves are dominant during strong sensory attention. Alpha and theta waves prevail during moods of diffuse attention or when attention is non-sensory and turned inward . . . As sleep deepens, delta waves become predominant. In deepest sleep the brain wave pattern is almost exclusively delta." (2, p. 203)

The discovery of Biofeedback has invalidated many long-held beliefs concerning the functioning of the autonomic (involuntary) nervous system. Researchers have had success in helping people control their blood pressure and heartbeat through the use of Biofeedback. It has also been effective in relieving stress-related conditions, especially migraine and tension headaches. An ever-increasing number of psychologists and psychiatrists are using Biofeedback in their treatments. Biofeedback is still in its infancy. More research is required before one will be able to accurately determine the limits of an individual's voluntary control over his body.

For more information on Biofeedback treatment in your area, contact your local psychologists and psychiatrists. For information concerning research programs and training, contact the colleges and universities in your vicinity or:

American Association of
Biofeedback Clinicians
2424 Dempster
Des Plaines, IL 60016

Additional reading:

1. Berkeley Holistic Health Center. *The Holistic Health Handbook.* Berkeley, CA: And/Or Press, 1978, p. 203.
2. *Brown, Barbara. *New Mind, New Body.* New York: Harper & Row, 1974.
3. Brown, Barbara. *Stress and the Art of Biofeedback.* New York: Harper & Row, 1977.
4. Jancks, Beata. *Your Body—Biofeedback at its Best.* Chicago: Nelson Hall, 1977.

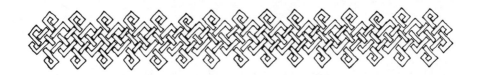

Hypnosis

The idea of hypnosis was first introduced to Western society by Anton Mesmer, a Viennese doctor. Mesmer presented his theories on hypnosis and "animal magnetism" to the French Court in the late 1700s. Later, when Mesmer's theories were discredited, the idea of hypnosis was abandoned for almost a century until a Scottish physician, Dr. James Braid, began to explore the uses of hypnosis in medicine. Dr. Braid is also responsible for coining the term "hypnosis" which he derived from *hypnos,* the Greek word for sleep. Freud, in his treatment of hysteria, was the first person to use hypnosis therapeutically. Since that time it has been widely used in psychotherapy. In 1959 the American Medical Association, recognizing the potential benefits to be derived from the use of hypnosis, named it an "adjunctive tool in medicine to be used with caution." Today hypnosis is a scientifically recognized and validated technique.

A state of hypnosis is produced through the suggestions of the hypnotist. The client concentrates totally on whatever suggestion the hypnotist uses to induce the hypnotic trance. A few typical examples of hypnotic suggestions are: Your eyelids are getting heavy, your right arm is becoming lighter and can float, and watch the pendulum. The purpose of the suggestion is to detach the client from her external environment and to get her to focus totally on what the hypnotist is saying. "The hypnotic state produced is by no means clear-cut. It is not an alpha state. It is not a state of 'rapid eye movement' (dreaming). It is not a state which can be delineated by any psychological measures. It is called a state only because it feels different from ordinary consciousness." (1, p. 242)

A trance is often described as being neither a waking nor a sleeping state of consciousness. In a trance one has the ability to function as if awake, but has no initiative to do so. A fundamental trait of a hypnotic state is that it produces a narrower, more highly focused range of attention. The depth of a trance is usually classified as a light, medium or deep state. "In *light hypnosis* the following symptoms can usually be produced: relaxation with a tendency not to move, inability to open eyelids, a general feeling of heaviness, and a partial age regression . . . In the *medium* depth of trance one experiences complete body catalepsy, anesthesia of any part of the body and control of some organic functions including bleeding and salivation . . . *Deep hypnosis* produces complete age regression, the ability to open one's eyes without awakening and complete anesthesia . . ." (4, p. 32)

Over the years hypnosis has been associated with quackery and as a result there are many popular misconceptions concerning its safety, the most common of these being that the client is under the hypnotist's power and that she can be made to do or say anything that the hypnotist wants. The truth of the matter is that during hypnosis a subject is never under the control of the hypnotist. The client is always aware of what she is doing or saying. No one can be made to do or say anything under hypnosis that is against her principles, nor will a client carry out a suggestion unless she feels it is acceptable. A viable alternative for an individual who is interested in gaining the benefits available through hypnosis, but who doesn't feel comfortable in going to a hypnotist, is self-hypnosis. Self-hypnosis, a method for mentally suggesting oneself into a trance, can easily be learned through books or classes. It is basically the same as hypnosis, although in some cases one is not able to go into as deep a trance as can be achieved when working with another person (a hypnotist).

Hypnosis, often thought of as the window to the mind, provides the easiest access to the subconscious—the area where the origins of one's psychological problems are stored. Through the various hypnotic techniques, the subconscious can be contacted and the roots of one's problems can be seen and understood. Hypnosis is now being used with success as a method for relaxation and for helping a person to overcome her negative behavior patterns such as overeating, smoking and drinking.

For more information about a professional hypnotist (physician, psychologist, psychiatrist or dentist) in your vicinity, contact:

> The Society for Clinical and Experimental
>   Hypnosis
> 265 West End Ave.
> New York, NY 10023
> (212) 873-7200

Additional reading:

1. Berkeley Holistic Health Center. *The Holistic Health Handbook.* Berkeley, CA: And/Or Press, 1978.
2. Bowers, Kenneth. *Hypnosis for the Seriously Curious.* Monterey, CA: Brooks/Cole, 1976.
3. Chauchard, Paul. *Hypnosis and Suggestion.* New York: Walker and Company, 1950.
4. Le Cron, Leslie. *Self-Hypnotism—The Technique and Its Use in Daily Living.* Englewood Cliffs, NJ: Prentice-Hall, 1964.
5. Ousby, William. *The Theory and Practice of Hypnotism.* New York: Arco, 1973.

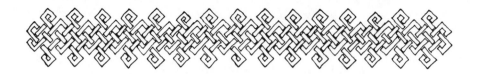

Silva Mind Control

Silva Mind Control (or psychorientology) is a method for increasing the powers of one's mind. It was created by Jose Silva for the purpose of teaching people how to gain control over certain brain functions that had previously been believed to be under the influence of the involuntary nervous system. Silva, the owner of an extremely successful electronics repair shop in Laredo, Texas, became very interested in the electrical impulses or wave functions of the brain. He believed that the lower brain wave states could be used to increase a person's capacity to recall information and to improve his IQ. After a great deal of study he began to experiment on his children. The results were so successful that neighbors requested he help improve their children's ability to study. During one such experiment with his daughter, she began to answer his questions before he had asked them. Not only that, she could tell him exactly, word for word, what the questions would be as they formed in his mind.

A large segment of Silva's research was devoted to finding the optimum brain wave frequency between the beta waves, which are associated with the alert state of mind, and the theta waves, which are indicative of deep sleep. Beta waves have a frequency of at least 14 cycles per second. Theta waves range from 4–7 cycles per second. Alpha waves are produced by the brain when it is functioning in the mid-range (7–13 cycles per second). The alpha state is often associated with the level of consciousness that meditators achieve while in meditation. It is with this range of awareness that Silva Mind Control works. Silva found that at this frequency people not only gained control of some of their involuntary biological functions such as heartbeat, blood pressure and blood circulation, but also were able to sense information that previously had been beyond them. Two of the most commonly experienced examples of these new powers are the ability to read someone else's mind and the ability to locate a missing object. At this point Silva switched the focus of his efforts from improving people's IQ's to training them to use their "effective sensory perception" while in the alpha state.

Once an individual has entered the alpha state, "the mind (master sense) can be projected to function from the alpha perspective and can be oriented to develop controls by establishing points of reference within the alpha dimension. The mind can learn to sense information impressed not only on its own alpha neurons but can sense information impressed on the alpha neurons of other brains regardless of distance." (1, p. 422)

Research has shown that the Silva Mind Control technique has been very useful in reducing stress and alleviating certain stress-related conditions, especially high blood pressure and headaches. Aside from being an aid to relaxation, it has also been effective in helping people overcome destructive habits such as overeating, smoking and drinking.

Since the classes formally began in 1966, over 500,000 people have taken the basic Silva Mind Control course. Two of the major factors responsible for its success are that 1) it is very easy to learn and 2) it does not require much practice. The basic course is comprised of four lectures, each requiring about ten hours of study. The lectures focus on two distinct forms of communication: 1) the objective and 2) the subjective. During the lessons on objective communication, a person learns to control undesirable habits, headaches, the relaxation of muscles, and how to improve his memory. The lessons on subjective communication teach an individual how to increase his effective sensory perception. One begins to develop personal reference points in the alpha dimension. In the final steps of the training a person learns how to project his mind in order to be able to read another person's mind, or locate a missing object.

There are Silva Mind Control centers in major cities throughout the world. For more information contact your local center or:

Silva Mind Control International, Inc.
1110 Snyder
Laredo, TX 78040
(512) 722-6391

Additional reading:

1. Matson, Katinka. *The Psychology Today Omni-book of Personal Development.* New York: William Morrow, 1977.
2. Silva, Jose, and Miele, Philip. *The Silva Mind Control Method.* New York: Pocket Books, 1977.

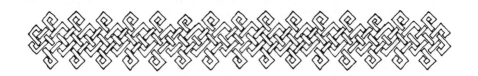

Autogenic Training

Autogenic Training (AT) is a method of self-hypnosis that leads to deep relaxation and greater powers of self-regulation, awareness and self-discovery. AT was developed by Dr. Johannes H. Schultz, a German physician, in 1929. Medical hypnosis in 1929 was by no means a new method of treatment. There was, however, until the advent of AT, no self-hypnotic technique that an individual could use proficiently. Dr. Schultz and his colleagues felt that a self-hypnotic method was required in order to lessen the dependence many clients had on their therapists. At the turn of the century (1900) a great deal of research was being done in the area of autohypnosis in an effort to devise a method which would enable a person to let herself in and out of a hypnotic trance at will. Out of this research Autogenic Training was born. Today AT is the most popular and widely accepted treatment for functional nervous diseases in Germany.

The motto as well as the goal of Autogenic Training can be summed up as "I am at peace." In order to achieve this goal, AT uses six exercises in which the client repeats silently one of the six standard AT phrases, while focusing her attention on the corresponding part of her body. An example of this is the first exercise: "My right arm is heavy." While concentrating on her right arm the client repeats the phrase a few times and then simply observes whatever emotions or feelings happen to arise. Every person's experience is unique and valid. It is soon discovered that through the use of these exercises an individual can learn to influence many bodily functions formerly believed to be controlled by the autonomic or involuntary nervous system. These functions, however, cannot be controlled at will; "only in a passive, concentrated state with an attitude of receptivity can one allow the desired functions to happen and thereby learn control of internal states." (1, p. 227)

In an AT session a hypnotic state of light trance is used. This is brought on through the repetition of the mood formula—"I am at peace." "The trance, a state of shallow hypnosis, is characterized by the seeking, attaining and remaining in an experiential level of diminished consciousness. The diminished consciousness of the trance-like state gives the subject the experiential field necessary to reach the goal of each exercise, as well as the specific quality of experience at this level of consciousness and the specific mode or relaxation." (2, p.5)

Once in the trance, the six basic phrases and visualization exercises are used. In a simplified form these are: "1) Right arm very heavy (for left-handed people, left arm); 2) Right (left) hand warm; 3) Pulse calm and strong; 4) Breath calm and clear; 5) Solar plexus glowing warm; 6) Forehead pleasantly cool." (2, p. xiii) These exercises, which should be practiced twice a day—twenty minutes at a time—reduce muscular tension, regulate and evenly distribute the blood flow throughout the body, and allow the biological activities such as respiration and heartbeat to find their own unforced pace. In short, AT produces feelings of profound well-being and total relaxation.

In addition to producing a state of tranquil relaxation, AT has been proven to be effective in the treatment of various stress-related diseases, including ulcers, high blood pressure, migraines and sexual problems. One can also learn to regulate habits such as overeating, drinking and smoking through the internal reprogramming of the idea that these habits are no longer important or conducive to good health.

Autogenic Training can be done in a group setting or individually. It is recommended that one begin the training with a properly certified instructor.

For more information contact:

Biofeedback Institute	Biofeedback Institute
3428 Sacramento St.	1800 N. Highland Ave.
San Francisco, CA 94118	Hollywood CA 90028
(415) 921-5455	(213) 462-8932

Additional reading:

1. Berkeley Holistic Health Center. *Holistic Health Handbook.* Berkeley, CA: And/Or Press, 1978.
2. Rosa, Karl. *You and AT.* New York: E.P. Dutton, 1973.
3. Shealy, Norman. *Autogenic Training.* New York: Dial Press, 1977.

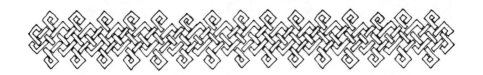

Selective Awareness Therapy

Selective Awareness Therapy is the method devised by Dr. Peter Mutke for creating a state of mind/body harmony. Dr. Mutke began his medical career as a general practitioner and surgeon in California. His growing interest in humanistic medicine led him to further study in the area of acupuncture, biofeedback and especially psychotherapy. Dr. Mutke is presently Professor of Psychology at John F. Kennedy University and the medical director of the Foundation for Humanistic Medicine. He is internationally known for his work with Selective Awareness.

Selective Awareness is a concentrated state of mind. Whenever an individual concentrates on anything, whether it be reading a book, watching TV or listening to music, he automatically screens out distracting stimuli. This state of focused attention is selective awareness. "If you were not in a state of selective awareness, you would not be able to concentrate on any one thing, because every bit of stimulus that reached you would be equally important and equally demanding of your attention." (1, p. 9)

Selective Awareness Therapy is based on the premise that a person is born with not only inherent self-healing powers, but a fundamental disposition towards health. If an individual's self-regulating process is functioning properly, he will be able to meet stress and changes to his internal (biochemical) and external environment without becoming ill. In order to maintain the homeostatic condition necessary for good health, a person must be in physiological and psychological harmony. When one's mind and body are not balanced, dis-ease results. Dr. Mutke writes, "Both physical and psychological symptoms are the product of unresolved thought-emotion complexes that upset your homeostatic balance by misallocation of energy. This misallocation of energy may actually cause illness. This means that how you think and what you feel influence your physical health. The reverse is also true—if you have a physical symptom for long, it will change the way you think and feel about everything else (the thought-emotion complex)." (1, p. 10)

Selective Awareness Therapy, a psychological self-care technique, is designed to facilitate mind/body integration by utilizing the principle of concentrated awareness to help an individual center attention on his areas of physical and/or mental imbalances. The stage of selective awareness attained in the therapy differs from the normal selective awareness that one experiences through the act of concentration. The therapy has been developed to use this power of concentration at a "higher" level—the alpha level. When an individual uses Selective Awareness Therapy, his brain wave pattern switches from the normal day-to-day activity pattern (beta wave) to the tranquil (alpha wave) pattern. The brain wave change is very therapeutic in and of itself, for it brings deep relaxation. Once in the alpha state, a person applies the various Selective Awareness Therapy exercises and techniques which enable him to contact the thoughts and feelings that lead to homeostasis. At this point one is then able to determine what changes have to be made in order to achieve mind/body harmony.

Selective Awareness Therapy, as stated earlier, is primarily a self-care technique. The exercises, which are easily mastered, can be learned from a therapist or through Dr. Mutke's book, *Selective Awareness*. Initially the time required to learn the exercises is approximately half an hour a day. Once mastered, the exercises can be used effectively in a shorter period of time wherever and whenever a person chooses. Selective Awareness Therapy has been shown to reduce tension and stress-related conditions such as headaches and high blood pressure. It has also been very effective in helping people to overcome undesirable habits including smoking, overeating and drinking. In addition to this, a large number of people have learned how to utilize their self-healing potential through the Selective Awareness Therapy techniques.

Additional reading:

1. Mutke, Peter H.C., M.D. *Selective Awareness.* Millbrae, CA: Celestial Arts, 1977.

body
therapies

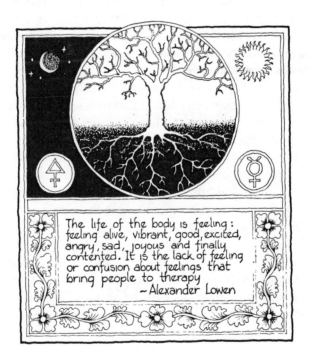

The life of the body is feeling:
feeling alive, vibrant, good, excited,
angry, sad, joyous and finally
contented. It is the lack of feeling
or confusion about feelings that
bring people to therapy
~ Alexander Lowen

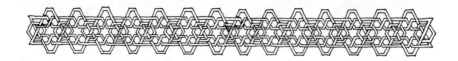

Massage

Massage is one of the oldest healing techniques known. Dating back to the earliest humans, massage has been used for centuries whenever people had physical pains, aches or bruises. "Massage as a term is used to designate certain manipulations of the soft tissue of the body. These manipulations are most effectively performed with the hands, and are administered for the purpose of producing effects on the nervous and muscular systems and the local and general circulation of the blood and the lymph." (1) Through the ages the various techniques of massage have been refined. Swedish massage, the most common method of massage used in Western society, was developed in the early part of the nineteenth century by Peter Ling. Ling traveled throughout Europe studying with many masseurs. The system of massage that he created incorporated many of the French techniques of stroking, kneading and pounding as well as his own methods of rolling, shaking, vibrating, and joint manipulations.

As the practice of medicine became increasingly more scientific and technical, the use of massage was neglected by doctors and became the province of physical therapists. In the recent past the art of massage has all but been abandoned. In the minds of many people, massage became associated with cheap massage parlors and prostitutes. At present, however, due to the human potential movement, the trend towards physical fitness, and increased awareness of the benefits of it, massage is experiencing a rebirth in popularity and acceptance.

Today there are many new massage schools and centers that practice only therapeutic massage techniques.* Massage has become a standard tool in the growing practices of sensory awareness and natural healing. The relaxing psychological aspects of massage as

---

*For information on therapeutic massage techniques, see the chapters on Shiatsu, Reflexology, Acupressure, Do-In, G-Jo, Rolfing, Lomi School, Postural Integration, and Polarity Therapy.

well as the release of muscular tension and cramps, the improvement of blood and lymph circulation, and the increased flexibility of one's joints make massage a highly pleasurable as well as healing experience.

For more information contact:

Esalen Institute
1756 Union St.
San Francisco, CA 94123

Esalen Institute
Big Sur, CA 93920

Acadia School of Massage
1220 North 45th St.
Seattle, WA 98103
(206) 632-8331

Northern California School of Massage and
    Natural Therapeutics
116 Elm St.
San Mateo, CA 94401
(415) 348-1034

Santa Fe Academy of Massage and Natural Healing
1590 Canyon Rd.
Santa Fe, NM 87501

Boulder School of Massage Therapy
P.O. Box 1881
Boulder, CO 80306
(303) 443-5131

Additional reading:

1. Beard, Gertrude. *Massage—Principles and Techniques.* Philadelphia: W. B. Saunders, 1964.
2. *Downing, George. *The Massage Book.* New York: Random House—Bookworks, 1972.
3. Hofer, Jack. *Total Massage.* New York: Grosset & Dunlap, 1978.

4. Inkela, Gordon, and Todris, Murray. *The Art of Sensual Massage.* New York: Simon & Schuster, 1972.
5. Leboyer, Frederick. *Loving Hands—The Traditional Indian Art of Baby Massage.* New York: Alfred A. Knopf, 1976.

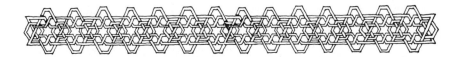

The following part of this section is devoted to the finger pressure massage therapies—Shiatsu, Do-In, G-Jo, Reflexology, and Acupressure. While it may seem that they are all alike, in reality they are actually quite different from each other. All of these therapies are similar in that they have been developed around the principle of stimulating the energy flow (Chinese Ch'i or Japanese Ki) in the body. However, each of the following techniques is different in not only the conceptual theory of how the energy circulates in the body, but also in how the actual technique is applied. Therefore a person who is trained in one of these disciplines is not necessarily proficient in another one of them.

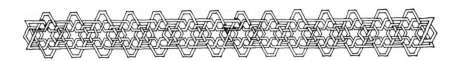

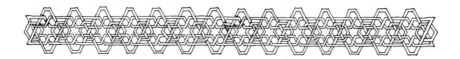

Shiatsu

Shiatsu is a Japanese form of finger pressure massage. The word Shiatsu is composed of the characters *shi*, meaning finger, and *atsu*, meaning pressure. It is a highly developed style of massage that is based on the proper application of the right amount of finger pressure on specific points throughout the body. Shiatsu is said to date back to the very beginning of human life, from the first time someone feeling either tired or in pain rubbed a part of his body. This natural reaction is considered to be both the true origin of and the key to Shiatsu. Practitioners of Shiatsu believe it is of the utmost importance to work with the body in as natural a way as possible. They believe that Shiatsu is able to work the wonders it does because it uses the natural reaction of the individual to press the ailing parts of the body in conjunction with taking advantage of the body's remarkable recuperative powers. Since its conception, a great deal of study and research has been done in order to scientifically systematize and improve this healing technique. While Shiatsu can and does cure many ailments, it is primarily a preventive measure which is used to keep the body in top physical shape so that conditions requiring medical attention will not develop.

This style of massage is done almost completely with the thumbs. Pressure is applied to any or all of the hundreds of Shiatsu pressure points located throughout the body. The pressure is usually held from five to seven seconds on all parts of the body except for the neck, where it is maintained for three seconds. The degree of pressure needed and used varies with the individual's symptoms, size and condition. A proficient Shiatsu therapist is able to apply pressure in a way that produces deep bodily changes without causing the client any discomfort. A Shiatsu treatment for a healthy person usually lasts about half an hour, while for an individual in poor condition it takes closer to an hour.

The pressure applied in a Shiatsu treatment stimulates the body's natural recuperative powers and rids the body of fatigue through the process of diffusing the carbon dioxide and lactic acid which when accumulated in the muscle tissue causes muscular stiffness and blood stagnation. The theory behind Shiatsu is that the body consists of 660 zones called *tsubo*. These areas, which are not visible, are the places where the "blood vessels, lymph vessels, nerves and ductless glands of the endocrine system tend to concentrate or branch out from." (2, p. 16) The tsubo are the areas of primary importance in the Shiatsu treatment. To truly facilitate the healing process, it is essential for the practitioner to not only know the exact location of the tsubo, but also how to vary the amount of pressure applied and how often each point should be stimulated.

Shiatsu is known to have many therapeutic effects, among them: 1) "Shiatsu stimulates the blood circulation and nourishment of the skin which in turn increases the ability of the skin to resist disease and infection. 2) The diffusion of the lactic acid and carbon dioxide in the muscle tissue due to the pressure of Shiatsu relieves muscular cramps and stiffness. 3) Shiatsu can help prevent nervous irregularities. When applied to the head Shiatsu stimulates the pituitary gland and the cerebral membrane which regulates the motor nerves and the nerves in charge of the memory and command functions to and from the brain. 4) Shiatsu helps to regulate the endocrine glands which are responsible for the secretion of the hormones. 5) The pressure used in Shiatsu stimulates the internal organs and helps to keep them functioning at their optimal level." (2, p. 16)

Shiatsu is not a difficult style of massage to learn. It is effective not only when given by one person to another, but it is also an excellent form of self-massage. After a short period of study one should be able to give his body a quick, effective "get your body going" massage in ten to fifteen minutes.

For more information contact:

Shiatsu Education Center of America
52 West 55th St.
New York, NY 10019
(212) 582-3424

Additional reading:

1. Namikoshi, Tokujiro. *Shiatsu Japanese Finger Pressure Therapy.* Tokyo: Japan Publications, 1972.
2. Namikoshi, Tokujiro. *Shiatsu Therapy Theory and Practice.* Tokyo: Japan Publications, 1974.

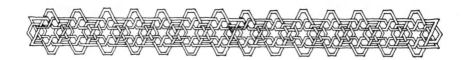

Do-In

Do-In, an ancient Chinese method of self-massage and breathing exercises, balances the Ki (breath) and helps to regulate an even, constant flow of energy through the meridians or energy pathways. Do-In is an esoteric science that had very few adherents in the West until Jacques deLangre's two books on the subject were published in the early 1970s. Mr. deLangre was himself introduced to the study of Do-In by Michio Kushi, the famous macrobiotic healer, author and teacher.

Do-In, which means "to lead with the breath," (2, p. 84) is believed to have been brought to China by Bodhidharma (Buddha) in order to help his monks improve their health and to keep their bodies attuned to the Tao, or natural flow of the Universe. Ki, the most important factor in the Do-In theory of the body and of the universe, is thought not only to be the breath and all that it entails such as the air and the life energy, but also is believed to be the dynamic energy which controls the interrelationship between *yin* and *yang*, the energies of action and inertia. It is also the name for the force which stimulates the internal organs and which binds all matter together electromagnetically. When Ki is present in the proper quantity and circulating freely through the body, one has good health. When there is an excess or a lack of Ki in the body, illness results.

Practitioners of Do-In believe that pain is most often created by excess stagnant energy in the afflicted area. At the same time there is a corresponding shortage of energy in another part of the body. By massaging the area where the excess has occurred, the energy is dispersed into the adjoining meridians, the same set of meridians and acupoints as used in acupuncture. The released energy is then able to circulate freely through the body to the area that has been suffering from a lack of energy. The freeing of the blocked energy allows the organs that are related to it through the sharing of a meridian to purify themselves through the renewed energy circulation. The essence of Do-In then, is to keep the Ki circulating freely through the body. When for some reason the Ki has become blocked, the practitioner of Do-In works with the body to free the energy and then lets the body heal itself through the use of its own energy. There are two fundamental massage techniques that are employed in the Do-In system to balance the Ki flow. "A deep and slow centrifugal spiral rotation of the thumbs" (1, p. 4) is used to calm and disperse excess energy. To stimulate an area which is acting sluggish due to a lack of energy, the fingertips are used in a series of light, rapid, superficial movements in the "shape of centripetal, concentric spirals." (1, p. 4)

The aim of Do-In is to allow an individual to live in the Tao—in true harmony with the natural order of the universe. In order to accomplish this it is very important to create the best environment to facilitate the optimal functioning of the Ki flow. This, the practitioners stress, cannot be accomplished simply by doing Do-In. Do-In, they feel, is a complementary treatment which is used most effectively when combined with a simple, natural diet, right livelihood and spiritual consciousness.

This system of self-massage consisting of a concise group of postures, breathing exercises and pressure points for stimulation is very easy to learn. While Do-In might not be able to bring one into the Tao on its own, it can be an effective form of preventive medicine. Starting each morning with a five minute Do-In self-massage is not only an invigorating way to begin the day, but a healthy one as well. Do-In used in this manner can help to point out any areas which may be sluggish or hyperactive. Once these areas have been identified, it can also be used to correct these imbalances which, if ignored, will lead to greater ailments. In cases where the individual might not be able to cure herself it can still be a useful tool for diagnosing a problem at an early stage in order to have it treated before it becomes harder to eliminate.

Additional reading:

1. deLangre, Jacques. *The First Book of Do-In.* Magalia, CA: Happiness Press, 1971.
2. deLangre, Jacques. *Second Book of Do-In.* Magalia, CA: Happiness Press, 1974.

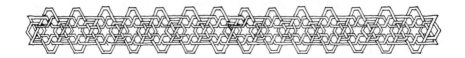

Reflexology—Zone Therapy

Reflexology, or Zone Therapy as it is often called, was brought to the attention of the Western medical world in 1913 by Dr. William H. FitzGerald. Dr. FitzGerald was a prominent physician, being at one point in his career the head of the Nose and Throat Department at St. Francis Hospital in Hartford, Connecticut. Although the principles of reflex massage had been known long before Dr. FitzGerald's time, they had been forgotten or passed over with the advance of modern medical technology. Dr. FitzGerald in his work rediscovered the healing powers of reflex massage and organized it in a way that made it more acceptable to Westerners—physicians and laypeople alike.

Reflexologists view the body as a unit composed of ten zones. The right and left sides of the body are the same and every zone runs not only vertically from the top of the head to the bottom of the feet, but also extends from the front to the back of the body. The theory upon which the reflexologists base their work is that everything in the body is represented in one of the ten zones. Each zone has a reflex area on both the hands and feet, which when massaged stimulates the various organs in that zone. To a proficient reflexologist the bottom of the feet as well as the hands are a map of the entire body with not only certain areas corresponding to each zone, but specific points for each and every organ in the body.

The feet play the central role in Reflexology, because it is believed that as the muscles in the body weaken, the muscle tissue in the foot is put under increasingly more strain, and it also weakens. As the body structure changes in this way undue pressure is put on one or more of the vast number of nerve endings in the feet. This results in the shutting off of part or all of the normal blood supply to that area of the foot which in turn slows down one's blood circulation. The decrease in blood circulation causes the formation of chemical deposits which hinder the circulation even more. This lack of free-flowing blood gives rise to many ailments, both major and minor, which are then expressed as sore areas on the feet.

Reflexologists believe that the circulation of the blood follows the flow of energy throughout the body. Thus, by stimulating the reflex points in the feet and hands, energy and blood are sent to those points and other areas in the affected zone. Through the practice of Reflexology it is possible to dissolve these crystals and bring the body's energy and blood circulation back to the proper level required for the body to heal itself.

The actual massage technique consists of using a "slow creeping rotary motion, not using the flat ball of the thumb as much as the corner toward the end." (2, p. 9) The amount of pressure applied should be as much as the client is able to endure. Reflexology is not always a soothing foot massage. For example, when the therapist is breaking up chemical deposits or is working on a point on the foot that corresponds to a weakness in the individual's body (example—the point for the lungs on a person who has asthma) it can be quite a painful experience. However, it is at these very times that Reflexology is the most beneficial not only as a means of improving one's health through an increase in blood and energy flow, but also as a diagnostic measure.

It is important to remember that the feet are accurate maps of the whole body and if a point on an individual's foot is sore then the corresponding part of his body is in a weakened condition. Using Reflexology as a guide to the areas which are not functioning optimally it is often possible to eliminate the problem before it requires a doctor's attention.

For more information contact:

Reflexology Institute
P.O. Box 1575
St. Petersburg, FL 33731

Additional reading:

1. Kaye, Anna, and Matchan, Don C. *Mirror of the Body.* San Francisco: Strawberry Hill Press, 1978.
2. Oliver, William H. *The Oliver Method of New Body Reflexology.* Provo, Utah: Bi-World Publishers, 1976.

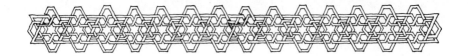

Acupressure

Acupressure is the Chinese form of healing which employs finger pressure massage on the acupuncture points. According to tradition the origin of acupuncture and acupressure dates back some five thousand years when "the Chinese noticed that pain could be relieved by rubbing stones against their bodies and that some soldiers, when wounded by arrows, recovered from long suffered illnesses." (2, p. 11) These occurrences led the Chinese to the idea that the stimulation of various points of the body is beneficial in the treatment of disease.

The theory underlying acupressure is very similar to that of Shiatsu, G-Jo, and the other Oriental massage techniques. The main principle of this theory is that disease is due to an imbalance in the flow of Ki (energy) throughout the body. By stimulating certain points as well as key combinations of points, the Ki flow is brought back into proper balance. When the energy is again able to circulate freely, the body is then able to heal itself. Acupressure does differ from the other schools of Oriental finger pressure massage in that it does not use the same points, although some may overlap, and the concept behind the theory is different. For example, a practitioner of Shiatsu views the body in terms of the 660 zones or tsubo, while a person using acupressure would look at the body in accordance with the acupuncture system of meridians and acupoints.

The technique used in acupressure is simple, harmless and quite effective. The massage itself is usually done with the thumb or index finger "in a small circular movement of two to three cycles per second." (2, p. 13) It is most effective when the pressure can be applied to both sides of the body (bilaterally) at the same time. The amount of time spent on stimulating any one point usually ranges from one to five minutes. The degree of pressure applied should be as much as the individual can comfortably tolerate.

Acupressure, like the other Oriental massage techniques, can be used to diagnose ailments as well as treat them. In addition to these uses it is probably most effective as a preventive measure. Through the use of acupressure in this manner one is able to keep her body in harmony and thus prevent or stop short many minor ailments that could normally lead to major diseases.

Additional reading:

1. Cerney, J. V. *Acupuncture Without Needles.* West Nyack, NY: Parker Publishing, 1974.
2. Chan, Pedro. *Finger Acupressure.* New York: Ballantine, 1974, p. 13.

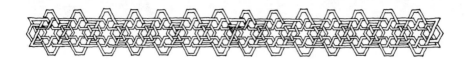

G-Jo

G-Jo is another Oriental massage technique that utilizes finger pressure stimulation of the acupoints for paramedical use. "G-Jo is a rough translation from Chinese meaning first aid." (1, p. xiii) First aid in China, however, is quite different from the first aid that most people in the West are accustomed to. In addition to the usual kinds of emergency treatment such as bandaging and splinting, Chinese first aid also encompasses keeping the body healthy through proper body maintenance, i.e. diet, exercise, and a positive mental attitude. In China there are thousands of "barefoot doctors" or paramedics who serve as a first line of medical care, treating people in their community who suffer from minor ailments. If a patient is too sick for, or not responding well to, the "barefoot doctors" treatment then he is sent to see a physician.

An important aspect of the "barefoot doctors" treatment is G-Jo. G-Jo rests on the same philosophy as acupuncture, acupressure, shiatsu and the other acupoint stimulation therapies. The essence of this philosophy is that the dis-ease is caused by an imbalance in the flow of the body's bioenergy, or what the Chinese call Ch'i. The imbalance in a person's bioenergy is thought to be due to an imbalance in his environment, either internally (mental, physical, emotional), externally or both. The first stage in correcting the irregularity then is to try to change the individual's lifestyle so that whatever was causing the energy imbalance can be eliminated. If, however, this cannot be done, the direct stimulation of the pressure points oftentimes can bring about the rebalancing of the Ch'i. This, in turn, will allow the body to complete its healing process. It is important to understand that in this system of medicine "good health means that bioenergy is flowing smoothly to the organs and that they are functioning properly; the 'mind' is peaceful and at one with the body. The person is relaxed, yet alert, and a controlled, positive energy seems to radiate from within." (1, p. xviii)

G-Jo is a style of finger pressure massage for basically healthy people who are interested in taking a more active part in their own health care. "Its goal is to temporarily relieve or reduce pain and symptoms of some disorders and illnesses." (1, p. 13) It can be used effectively on oneself or on other people as well. The technique itself is again similar to that of the other finger pressure massage techniques. After locating the proper point one should use his fingertip to stimulate it. The actual motion is circular—it should be "deep, tight, brisk and done in a counterclockwise direction for fifteen to twenty seconds." (1, p. 5) Unless the point lies on the spine or on the frontline meridian, it is important to stimulate the corresponding point on the other side of the body. The thumb is often used in cases where more pressure is needed than can be exerted with the fingertips.

G-Jo is the simplest of all the finger pressure massage techniques to learn. There are seven essential or most commonly used points, none of which are difficult to locate and the proper movement is easy to master. The G-Jo system was virtually unknown in the West until Michael Blate published *The G-Jo Handbook* in 1976. In this concise, easy to read and follow book one will find everything he needs to begin to learn G-Jo and to begin taking a more active role in his own health care.

Additional reading:

1. Blate, Michael. *The G-Jo Handbook*. Davie, Florida: Falkynor Books, 1976.

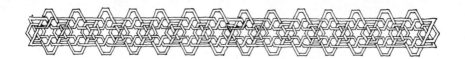

Touch For Health

Touch For Health is a system of health care that employs muscle testing, applied muscle kinesiology, acupressure and massage in order to improve postural balance and reduce physical and mental pain and tension. Dr. John Thie, a chiropractor, developed the Touch For Health system and packaged it in the form of a workbook and class instruction that makes this system of applied muscle kinesiology easily understandable and of practical use to laypeople as both a diagnostic tool and a very valuable preventive measure. This system is rooted in the work of another chiropractor, Dr. George Goodheart, who in the early 1960s began working with the then-new idea that the underlying cause of muscle spasms and pains which pulled the spine out of alignment was weak muscles on one side of the spine. The weak muscle causes the corresponding antagonistic muscle on the other side of the spine to become tight in order to counterbalance the weakness. This, in turn, produces muscle pain and spasms as well as resulting in the spine being pulled out of the proper alignment.

Built upon this basic premise, the Touch For Health system uses muscle testing as a diagnostic tool to determine both the need for a treatment and the effectiveness of the treatment after it has been given. Muscle testing is the process of isolating individual muscles apart from their supporting or synergistic muscles—muscles that ordinarily assist in any given movement. Once the muscle has been isolated, its strength is tested by pushing against the muscle in a specific direction while the individual resists.

The theory underlying Touch For Health is that good health comes from within. The two important prerequisites for good health are 1) good posture and 2) a well-balanced relationship between the different segments of the body. The awareness of the extreme importance of the interrelationships between the various parts of the body gives rise to the idea of holistic healing. This concept is crucial in

Touch For Health, for while the focus of the work is concentrated on correcting specific muscle weaknesses, it does not just treat the muscles, but the whole body. Practitioners of Touch For Health view the body as a highly integrated unit. Anything that affects one segment or part of this unit, no matter how small, will have an effect upon the entire unit, for the body as a whole will have to compensate for the change that has taken place in it. In Touch For Health theory some muscles are more closely related to one organ than to others through the sharing of an acupuncture meridian or a lymph vessel. When the muscle has been improved through the restoring of the proper energy flow to these meridians or energy pathways, the organs which share them will also benefit. An example of this inter-relationship between all the systems in the body is the following.

> If there is a tight muscle in the hip from a corresponding weakness on the opposite side, then the hip is favored because of the tension restricting its motion. That puts a different strain on the foot, and with the foot in a different position, there will be a strain on other sets of muscles. This is going to change the body's general posture, affecting the position of the internal organs. That in turn restricts the nutrition to the organs and changes the excretions and hormonal functions. The psychobiological/chemical balance of the person is changed and this affects the individual cells in the body. As the body and mind are affected the person will think and feel differently, so he/she is going to assume still a different posture. Then there is one more tight area, one more tension, one more cycle. So everything done affects all the rest. (1, p. 7)

Muscle testing forms the core of the Touch For Health system. Using these tests, the practitioners are able to evaluate both the function of the muscle and the effectiveness of the treatment on the muscles they are working with. The performance of the muscle is based on how well it is able to contract. Each individual's optimal level of strength varies as to her body size, but there should be no more than a 15% difference between the right and left sides regardless of which hand the person uses most often. The muscle test does more than indicate whether or not the muscle needs treatment. If the muscle is found to be weak or painful upon testing, it means that not only is that specific muscle in a weakened condition, but also any organ that shares the energy pathway with it. In the case that a muscle does need treatment, the practitioners most often use acupressure massage to drain the lymphatics which frequently become blocked with toxins, light contact and stroking of the acupuncture meridians to balance the energy flow, as well as muscle massage at the points of muscle attachments. Depending upon how the muscle has responded to the treatment, nutritional and/or herbal remedies may be suggested to help bring the muscle back up to par.

In summary, the Touch For Health system tests muscles for their relative strengths. Those that are found to be weak are strengthened by the techniques mentioned above. When the major muscles are of equal or near-equal relative strength, posture is improved, the energy flow is balanced and normal body functioning is permitted.

For more information contact:

Touch For Health Foundation
P.O. Box 751 C
1174 N. Lake Ave.
Pasadena, CA 91104
(213) 794-1181

Additional reading:

1. Thie, John, D.C., with Marks, Mary. *Touch For Health*. Santa Monica, CA: DeVorss & Company, 1973.

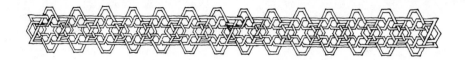

Polarity Therapy

Polarity Therapy is a complete system of health care utilizing diet, exercise, physical manipulation and proper mental attitude for attaining and maintaining good health. Dr. Randolph Stone, an extremely gifted and dedicated man, is the creator of Polarity Therapy. Born in Austria in 1890, Dr. Stone immigrated to the United States at the age of 13. As a young man he began his studies of Western science and natural healing, becoming a naturopath, chiropractor and osteopath. At the age of twenty-four he was awarded a special "Other Practitioners" license by the State of Illinois, which allowed him to practice not only the techniques that he had studied, but also to use other therapies from the entire field of drugless medicine. Feeling that the Western view of the body, health and illness was incomplete, he began to study the traditional medical practices of other cultures. This research led to years of extensive travel and study all over the world. During this time he became primarily interested in the medical systems of the East, especially acupuncture, Chinese herbal medicine, and the Ayurvedic and yogic healing methods of India. In 1948 Dr. Stone wrote *Energy: The Vital Principle in the Healing Art* in which he laid out the framework of Polarity Therapy. For the twenty-five years following the publication of his book, Dr. Stone focused his attention on his private practice while continuing to expand and refine the principles of Polarity. The system of Polarity that is used today is a unique synthesis of Eastern and Western techniques which he organized and developed over his sixty-year career. Dr. Stone retired in 1973 at the age of 83 to India, where he currently lives.

The fundamental principle in Polarity is that of energy. In Polarity theory energy is considered the basic ingredient of life. Dr. Stone believes that underlying everything in the physical (material) world is an infinite amount of universal energy. The term Polarity is derived from the concept that everything in the universe has two electrical poles (negative and positive) and that energy flows between them as in the case of the north and south poles of a magnet. This theory is also represented in the Chinese philosophy of yin-yang. Dr. Stone thought that energy in the body was transformed within the *chakras* (subtle body energy centers) of the body, and that once transformed it was then able to be used for specific life functions. Each chakra corresponds to one of the five basic elements (ether, air, fire, water, earth) of life. Life force energy is created when energy is united with these five elements. *Ether* is associated with the higher chakras; communication, psychic awareness, spirituality, throat and head. *Air* corresponds to the heart chakra; respiration, compassion, lungs and heart. *Fire* is related to the upper belly chakra (above the navel); digestion and assimilation, will and power, stomach and intestines. *Water* is linked to the pelvic/genital chakra; reproduction, emotional drive, liquid elimination and glandular secretions. *Earth*, the root chakra, is associated with physical survival, solid elimination, the rectum and the base of the spine.

Dr. Stone believes that an important characteristic of life energy is the *triune function.* He explained the triune function as that state in a living organism where the energy is balanced and flowing freely between the positive and negative electrical poles. When this occurs a neutral charge is produced. The triune function is the continual free flow of positive-neutral-negative energy. According to Polarity theory it is of the utmost importance for an individual's energy to be balanced, for only when the triune function is operating effectively is one able to be in the state of harmony required for good health.

The Polarity system treats a person in a holistic manner. Practitioners of Polarity believe that the physical, mental, emotional and spiritual aspects of a person's being are always in a dynamic (ever fluctuating) state. Furthermore, these different components of oneself are seen to be not different between themselves, but different manifestations of the same energy. An example of this is that an emotional problem which blocks the free flow of energy for a period of time will eventually lead to a physical ailment. "Therefore, in order to bring an individual into harmony with himself it is appropriate to give attention to whatever aspects of the person seem to be unbalanced, even if there is not (yet!) a crisis level of disease." (1, p. 101)

Keeping in mind the unity of the body, Dr. Stone created a far-reaching four-part integral system of therapy that is capable of treating an individual in a complete manner. The four segments of Polarity are 1) *Diet,* essentially fresh fruits, vegetables and some grains. No meat, fish, eggs, alcohol or drugs. Dr. Stone also developed a number of special diets and recipes to aid people involved in various types of cleansing processes. An example of this is the "liver flush," a drink that is effective in helping to restore and cleanse the kidneys and the intestinal tract. 2) *Exercise*—Polarity Yoga, a series of exercises specifically designed by Dr. Stone to facilitate the opening of physical and energy blocks in the body. 3) *Polarity manipulation*— the Polarity system of body work was developed out of Dr. Stone's vast knowledge of chiropractic, osteopathic and Oriental massage techniques. The touch (or technique) used is very similar to that of acupressure. However, the actual points and map of the body are unique to Polarity Therapy. It is a complete system of body work in that it includes methods for dealing with all types of energy imbalances whether they are physical, emotional or any other kind. 4) *Right Attitude*—Dr. Stone was a firm believer in the theory that most physical ailments were due to blocked emotional and mental energy. In order to alleviate problems of this nature, Polarity therapists stress the importance of maintaining a good mental attitude. In order to encourage this they employ techniques such as affirmations, which help build up an individual's positive feelings about herself. Typical examples of the affirmations used are: I am a good person, I am a smart and capable individual, I feel love for myself and others, etc. In summary, Polarity Therapy is a complete and powerful method of holistic healing that utilizes diet, exercise, physical manipulation and proper mental attitude in an interdependent manner in order to help an individual reach and maintain her optimum level of health.

There are at present two schools of Polarity Therapy. Upon his retirement in 1973, Dr. Stone appointed Pierre Pannetier, a student of his for ten years, to be his successor. Pannetier is the director of the Polarity Therapy Center in Orange, California. Dr. Stone also gave permission to Jefferson Campbell to use Polarity in conjunction with the Gestalt techniques he had learned as a student of Fritz Perls at Esalen. Campbell established his school, the Polarity Health Institute in Olga, Washington. While both men adhere closely to Dr. Stone's teachings, the body work done at the Polarity Health Institute uses a deeper or harder "touch" than the physical manipulations done at Pannetier's Polarity Therapy Center.

For more information contact:

> Polarity Therapy Center
> 401 North Glassell
> Orange, CA 92666
>
> Polarity Health Institute
> P.O. Box 86
> Olga, WA 98279
> (206) 376-2291

Additional reading:

1. Berkeley Holistic Health Center. *The Holistic Health Handbook.* Berkeley, CA: And/Or Press, 1978.
2. Stone, Randolph. *Energy: The Vital Principle in the Healing Art.* Chicago: Private Printing, 1948.

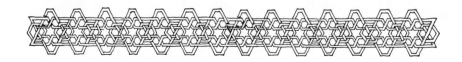

Alexander Technique

Considered by many to be the original mind/body therapy and the forerunner to the other such disciplines mentioned in this book, the Alexander Technique has been from its inception revolutionary in its approach to the problem of reeducating people to use their bodies in a more constructive manner. Frederick Matthias Alexander was born in Australia in 1869. A devotee of the theater, Alexander became a recitationist and actor. It was at this time he encountered the problem that was to lead him to his life's work. During recitals he would often lose his voice for no apparent reason. When his doctor could not help him, Alexander began to observe carefully how he used his body while speaking. In this period, which lasted almost ten years, he discovered that the key to his disability was "a very slight, all but imperceptible, yet seemingly inveterate accompaniment to every movement he made: a dismaying tendency to pull his head backwards and downwards. The prevention of this involuntary constraint, he found, lay in a technique of physical reeducation based upon a certain dynamic relationship of the head, neck and torso." (1, p. xiii) For the remaining sixty years of his life, Alexander dedicated himself to teaching his principles of body reeducation. He had many famous students and supporters over the years, including H. G. Wells, Aldous Huxley, John Dewey, George Bernard Shaw and Fritz Perls.

The Alexander Technique is designed to help people use their bodies more efficiently and with greater ease. Alexander believed that throughout one's life a person develops many patterns of movement which cause excessive fatigue and tension while also contributing to bad posture. He felt that over time people grow so accustomed to their habitual patterns of movement that no matter how uncoordinated or inefficient they have become, they still feel right. Through the Alexander Technique the student is helped to change his movement patterns. Alexander discovered that all of an individual's movements, from the most strenuous to the simplest, require complex patterns of movement which result in the particular way that the person uses himself. Alexander insisted that each movement, no matter how small, involved "the whole integrated (psychophysical) person." (1, p. xxiii) He believed the prerequisite of good movement was that the spine should be lengthened to the greatest extent possible in whatever movement is being undertaken. This lengthening of the vertebrae in activity he called "the true and primary movement in each and every act." (1, p. xxiii) In order to bring this into effect he developed the basic Alexander Technique of "primary control." This technique focuses on the specific relationship of the head and neck which allows an individual to achieve and maintain proper body use. An oversimplified description of the technique is: "let the neck be free, let the head go forward and up, and let the torso lengthen and widen out." (1, p. xxiv)

The Alexander lessons are based on teaching the student how to develop and maintain "primary control." The Alexander Technique differs from most other movement awareness disciplines in that the student is required "to make a conscious decision to do nothing. This of course does not mean the student remains in an immobile state." (1, p. xxvii) The student, after becoming conscious of his bad movement patterns, is taught how to "inhibit" them. This is done through a process where the Alexander teacher presents the student with a series of verbal directions such as sit, stand or walk. The student's role is to work at learning how to "consciously refuse to make the involuntary preparations or 'sets' that he has always made before performing such actions." (1, p. xxvii) For example, tensing the calf muscles before standing up. The teacher also describes what movements should take place and while the student repeats the instructions to himself the teacher helps to guide him through these new movement patterns.

The goal of the Alexander Technique is to replace the old habits with the improved movement patterns. When this is accomplished, the body alignment changes—the head moves up from the top of the spine; the spine lengthens to relieve abnormal curves and pressures; the musculature supporting the skeletal frame is neither contracted nor relaxed, but is dynamically balanced.

The Alexander Technique has been used for years as a valuable method to help people use their bodies with maximum ease and effectiveness. Among those who have often turned to the Alexander

Technique are many actors, actresses, dancers and singers, as well as those whose posture is bad or uncomfortable.

For more information contact:

> The American Center for the Alexander
>   Technique, Inc.
> 142 West End Ave.
> New York, NY 10023
> (212) 799-0468

> The American Center for the Alexander
>   Technique, Inc.
> 931 Elizabeth St.
> San Francisco, CA 94114

> The American Center for the Alexander
>   Technique, Inc.
> 812 Seventeenth St.
> Santa Monica, CA 90403
> (213) 451-3641

Additional reading:

1. Alexander, Frederick M. *The Resurrection of the Body*. New York: Dell, 1974.
2. Alexander, Frederick M. *Constructive Conscious Control of the Individual*. New York: E. P. Dutton, 1923.
3. Alexander, Frederick M. *The Use of the Self*. New York: E.P. Dutton, 1932.
4. Alexander, Frederick M. *The Universal in Constant Living*. New York: E. P. Dutton, 1941.
5. Barlow, Wilfred. *The Alexander Technique*. New York: Alfred A. Knopf, 1973.

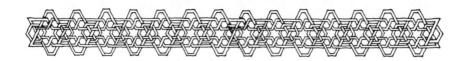

Feldenkrais Method

The Feldenkrais Method of movement awareness is the highly effective, scientifically based work of Dr. Moshe Feldenkrais. Dr. Feldenkrais emigrated from Russian Poland to Palestine as a young
man and later went to France, where he received his doctorate in
physics and became an associate of the famous Joliot-Curie. Aside
from his interest in physics, Dr. Feldenkrais was an outstanding
athlete in his youth. He holds a black belt in judo and was an ardent
soccer player. It was a soccer injury to his knee that decided his fate.
In 1940 he was informed by a surgeon whom he had consulted that
an operation which should have been performed on his knee years
before would now have only a fifty-fifty chance of success. Not lik-
ing the odds, Feldenkrais decided that he would teach himself to
walk all over again, which he did. In order to do this he studied anatomy, physiology, psychology and anthropology. Out of this intense period of study, his inquiries into different schools of yoga and
his perceptions of what the books neglected to teach him evolved his
own original method of human awareness through movement. At
present Dr. Feldenkrais is the Director of the Feldenkrais Institute in
Tel Aviv, a lecturer at the Hebrew University and at age seventy-five
the author of sixteen books.

The goal of the Feldenkrais Method is to break down one's habitual patterns of movement and behavior and replace them with
awareness and the ability to be spontaneous. Dr. Feldenkrais believes that what makes a human being essentially different from any
other animal is the functioning of her nervous system. "While animal
instinct is phylogenetic learning—or the learning of the species,
human learning is ontogenetic, i.e. it needs personal experience. In
short, learning is to the human nervous system what instinct is to an
animal." (1, p. 21) A person's ability to constantly learn and develop
new responses to stimuli is a crucial factor in her growth as an individual. "The human nervous system in which the patterns of actions

71

are wired in during the learning process and are not inherited (as are instincts) has a major advantage: relearning or reeducation is comparatively easy." (1, p. 1) It is this process of reeducation which Dr. Feldenkrais is concerned with.

At the present time, in the so-called normal course of human development, most people's coordination has become impaired by the age of three. An individual is likely to have noticeable bodily and postural defects by the time she has gone through adolescence. "The body is already twisted, tilted and rigid in some positions. At this point the individual has lost awareness of his body image (the body's surface and the joints of the skeletal structure) to the extent that his actions become more and more automatic, and patterns of muscular tension have developed of which he has little or no consciousness." (3, p. 42) A vital step in the reeducation process is to restore this awareness, for until a person regains body awareness it is impossible to determine what is the best way to use herself.

In order to break down the habitual patterns of movement which will lead to the restoration of awareness, a change in the dynamics of an individual's reactions is required. This cannot be achieved by merely replacing one action by another. Such a change demands a change of one's self-image which Feldenkrais states is "composed of four components that are involved in every action: movement, sensation, feeling and thought." (1, p. 31)

Central to the Feldenkrais technique is the idea of the unity of thought, feeling and movement. No thought, emotion or sensation of any kind is possible without a corresponding change in the musculature of the body. Similarily, changes in the configuration of muscular patterns necessarily activate patterns of thought, emotion and sensation. In short the whole nervous system participates in every act. Since any of the four components of the waking state (movement, sensation, thought and feeling) inescapably influence the others, a change in any one can be used to break the habitual behavior patterns.

Dr. Feldenkrais chose to work with movement as his force for change, because "it is easier to distinguish the quality of a movement than a thought or emotion." (1, p. 38) The Feldenkrais Method is designed to help bring about a better maturation of one's nervous system. This is accomplished through establishing or reestablishing connections between the motor cortex and the musculature that have been short-circuited due to tension, bad habits, psychological or environmental influences. The final aim is a body that is organized to move with minimum effort and maximum efficiency, not through increased muscular strength or flexibility, but through an increase in the consciousness of how the body functions.

The Feldenkrais Method is composed of two parts, the manipulative technique or "hands on" type of body work called Functional Integration, and a series of movement lessons termed Awareness Through Movement. Functional Integration is an individual technique in which the Feldenkrais instructor custom tailors the treatment to fit the particular needs of each client. These sessions are very helpful for gaining a more in-depth awareness of the problem areas of one's body. The Awareness Through Movement lessons which use exercises as opposed to body work were created to produce the same effect as Functional Integration, only in a larger number of people. Today in most cases a person involved in the Feldenkrais Method would spend the majority of her time in a group doing the Awareness Through Movement lessons and would have Functional Integration treatments periodically on the problem areas of her body. The exercises which are done in a group are extremely relaxing and never goal oriented.

The lessons are done in the lying position, prone or supine, to facilitate the breakdown of muscular patterns and to neutralize the effect of gravity. "The lessons are performed slowly and as pleasantly as possible with absolutely no pain or strain at all. The movements are very light, so that after fifteen or twenty repetitions the initial effort drops to practically nothing more than a thought. This produces the maximum sensitivity in the person and enables her to detect the minute changes in the efferent tonus and the change in the alignment of the different parts of the body." (1, p. 31) Throughout the Awareness Through Movement classes one constantly hears, "If it hurts don't do it" and "Never do more than you can do, given the limits of pleasure." These instructions given with virtually every movement are extremely important, for they allow the mind to release from its habitual response of "If I push myself I can do it." A by-product of relaxing and working with one's body is almost always a surprising achievement far beyond that which one had previously thought possible. This kind of performance is the key to the Feldenkrais teachings which Dr. Feldenkrais aptly sums up as "If you know what you do, you can do what you want."

At the last count Dr. Feldenkrais had a repertoire of over one thousand lessons which he has devised and used in his work. "Repeatedly as all kinds of movements are performed, the awareness is continually directed to the body and the change resulting from the various movements. Over time this leads to a feeling of lightness, an ease of movement, an expansion of awareness and a body-mind oriented to and capable of a greater range of experience." (3, p. 48)

For more information contact:

Esalen Institute
Big Sur, CA 93920

Additional reading:

1. Feldenkrais, Moshe. *Awareness Through Movement.* New York: Harper & Row, 1972.
2. Feldenkrais, Moshe. *Body and Mature Behavior.* New York: International Universities Press, 1970.
3. Master, Robert. "The Feldenkrais Method." *Saturday Review,* February 22, 1975.

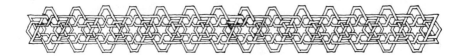

Aston–Patterning

Aston–Patterning, a movement education system, is designed to help people use their bodies in a more efficient manner. Students of Aston–Patterning often describe this increased efficiency in terms such as having more energy, more vitality and increased emotional well-being. Many students have reported improved physical health and appearance.

Judith Aston, the originator of Aston–Patterning, has an impressive background in movement education. She was the movement facilitator with the San Diego Gestalt Institute and worked with Dr. Ida P. Rolf as the director of the Structural Patterning Institute, which uses patterning in conjunction with Structural Integration.

The goal of Aston–Patterning is to enable a person to move with ease in ways that best reflect the mind's intentions. Aston practitioners believe that all movement reveals a pattern, and that these patterns may be in either conflict or harmony with an individual's true expression. The need for patterning arises when one or more of the body segments moves out of balance or vertical alignment. This movement out of alignment is most commonly caused by stress or injury. As this shift off the center occurs, all of the other body segments must adjust in placement or tension in order to counterbalance it. In order to maintain this imbalance, new movement patterns are needed. Once the repetition of these movements has become habitual, the new off-center patterns are locked into the individual's structure. Through the use of patterning, students are able to get in touch with the inner wisdom of their bodies and thus are able to better express their well-proportioned selves. An additional benefit derived from Aston–Patterning is the centering of the mind, for as the body moves into better balance so does the mind.

This approach, which usually consists of about twelve lessons, entails a gradual, step-by-step process of changing one's movement patterns. The practitioners realize that the proper pattern of alignment for everyone is unique; thus each lesson is especially tailored to the person's specific needs. Through these techniques the student is able to learn about the patterns that he has been holding on to, whether they are mental (holding out for what he thinks is the ideal situation), emotional (holding back his feelings) or physical (holding on to tension). There are an infinite number of ways to hold patterns and just as many reasons for doing so, but when energy is unnecessarily spent repeatedly holding imbalanced patterns, then the individual's body begins to take a distorted shape due to these stressful patterns which are in conflict with whom the person actually is.

During the lessons the teacher helps the student become aware of the way he is using his body in ordinary, everyday situations such as standing, sitting and walking. Once the student has become aware of the movement patterns he is using, the patterner then guides the individual in more healthful and graceful ways of moving while engaged in these activities. As the student's awareness increases, the patterner continues to lead him in finding more beneficial movement patterns in the specific areas of his interest whether it be construction work, tennis, or better driving posture.

For more information contact:

The Aston–Patterning Institute
P.O. Box 114
Tiburon, CA 94920
(415) 435-0433

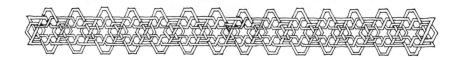

Dance Therapy

Dance Therapy is the use of dance as an instrument to bring about the integration of the physical and emotional aspects of an individual. Marian Chace was the originator of Dance Therapy. A dancer with the Denishawn Company in the late 1930s, she was also an avid student of the traditional dances of other cultures. In her own dance school in Washington, D.C., Chace focused her attention on the students as individuals instead of the structure or form of the dance. Due to her unconventional approach, her students often felt that her dance classes provided them with the opportunity to release tension and gain a sense of emotional well-being that they had not previously experienced. In 1942 the psychiatrists at St. Elizabeth's Hospital in Washington, D.C., were investigating new methods of group therapy. They invited her to begin the first experimental program in Dance Therapy. The program was an immediate success. Dance Therapy was found to be an especially effective means of dealing with clients who for one reason or another were not verbally communicative. Until the 1960s, Dance Therapy was considered mainly an adjunctive therapy. With the advent of the human potential movement, Dance Therapy has grown in acceptance and is now seen as a primary form of therapy by many therapists and physicians. In 1966 The American Dance Therapy Association was established.

Dance Therapy is founded on the belief that physical movement is not only a fundamental medium for self-expression but a primary and basic means of communication. The physical body is seen as a reflection of an individual's internal feelings. The way that he moves is viewed as an expression of those internal feelings. In accordance with this philosophy, Dance Therapy considers a realistic body image and mind/body integration to be basic ingredients for good mental health. The dance therapist's work is aimed at helping a person to achieve this mind/body integration. In order to accomplish this the therapist encourages the client to become freer and more flowing in his movements. As the movements begin to open up or expand, the unlocking of the rigid musculature begins to take place. "A body with a tensely locked musculature can only make incomplete, clonic movements. These movements cannot send clear signals to the brain since the synapses which pass on nervous impulses remain closed. Only the complete tonic movements of a healthy, aligned body can promote a free system of communication between body and brain. The dance therapist works at making a patient's gestures and movements strong, meaningful, larger than life, in order to open the 'locked' synapses." (1, pp. 132-133) The opening up of the constricted body through movement allows one to experience a significant emotional release as well as a healthy means of "blowing off" tension.

Dance Therapy can be done individually or in group sessions. Group sessions are usually preferred in that they encourage a person to express himself to a greater degree through the initiation of group movement.

For more information contact:

American Dance Therapy Association
10400 Connecticut Ave., Suite 300
Kensington, MD 20795
(301) 997-4040

Dance Notation Bureau
505 Eighth Ave.
New York, NY 10018
(212) 736-4350

Additional reading:

1. Lefco, Helene. *Dance Therapy—Narrative Case Histories of Therapy Sessions with Six Patients.* Chicago: Nelson-Hall, 1974.
2. Rosen, Elizabeth. *Dance in Psychotherapy.* New York: Dance Horizons Publications, 1974.

mind body therapies

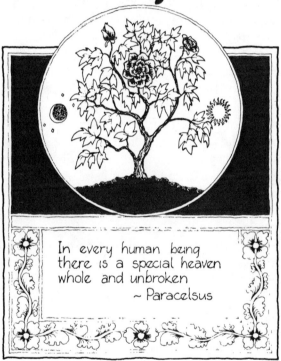

In every human being
there is a special heaven
whole and unbroken
                ~ Paracelsus

Structural Integration

Structural Integration, or Rolfing, as it is popularly known, is a mind/body discipline which has evolved from the work of Dr. Ida P. Rolf. Dr. Rolf was an organic chemist with the Rockefeller Institute who spent many years researching Structural Integration before developing this program.

Structural Integration is a systematic technique for restructuring the body through deep tissue manipulation so as to bring its major segments—the head, thorax, shoulders, pelvis and legs into a more vertical alignment in order to give the individual better balance in both stance and movement. This in turn creates a more efficient relationship between the individual and the field of gravity. Gravity, a key force in the theory of Structural Integration, is not believed by Rolfers (practitioners of Structural Integration) to be the negative force that many people feel it is—pulling them downward and causing discomfort. Gravity becomes damaging when one or more of the body segments move out of the vertical alignment. At this point both the skeleton and musculature are forced into an inefficient weight-bearing function. This creates resistance to gravity which is the destructive factor. The goal, then, is to realign a person in a way that enables her body to have the most harmonious relationship possible with the field of gravity.

The Rolfing treatment itself is a series of ten sessions, each lasting approximately one hour and usually scheduled at least a week or more apart. In these sessions the Rolfer works at rebalancing the fascial tissue through the use of deep pressure massage techniques. Fascial tissue is the tissue that envelops and connects muscles to one another. Inefficient and negative physical behavior patterns become set over a period of time in the fascial network and are manifest as unbalanced patterns of structure. The theory behind Structural Integration is that by reordering the fascial tissue the structural imbalances will be removed; thus the body can be properly aligned.

The first seven sessions are spent on opening up and relieving the local areas of contraction and imbalance in order to make the body more fluid. In the last three sessions the work centers around putting the body back together in proper alignment. More specifically, in the first three sessions the opening up process is begun on the surface layers of the body. In sessions four through six the work is continued on the deeper levels of the body. Session seven is usually reserved for work on the face. The last three sessions focus on using the new fluidity in the body to properly integrate the major segments of the new structure and to get the person to function well as a whole body. Research conducted at Agnews State Hospital in California has shown that Structural Integration, aside from improving the posture and circulation, also increases muscle efficiency, thus allowing the individual to conserve energy.

Structural Integration is often a painful experience. The pain is sometimes tied into emotional repression that is causing inner tensions and resistance. In these instances the pain, which is due to the resistance to the Rolfer's stimulation of the bound (contracted or displaced) area, triggers both an emotional as well as a physical release. The Rolfer oftentimes helps to guide the emotional release by having the individual use various breathing or Gestalt techniques.

In many cases people think of Rolfing or the other disciplines based on similar principles of deep connective tissue massage (Lomi Body Work and Postural Integration) only in terms of being painful experiences, which they don't feel they can handle or at least don't care to try. Being Rolfed is a very personal experience which is hard to put into words. Each individual's body is so unique that the range of sensations one goes through during the Structural Integration process is only understandable to that individual. In many cases there aren't even words in our language to accurately describe these feelings. Some people might not find it very painful while others may find it excruciating. This might be true for the whole ten sessions or on a session-to-session basis. The pain itself is not a lasting pain and it does stop as soon as the Rolfer releases the pressure. In summary, if the only reason one chooses not to get involved with a deep connective tissue massage therapy is because she is concerned about the pain involved, then it is recommended that the individual talk to a practitioner of the discipline of her interest. One might well be surprised how easily the discomfort can be borne and how glad she is to do it for the benefits received.

The long-range physical effects of Rolfing vary greatly from individual to individual, depending upon how much effort the individual makes in trying to use her new structure properly. In order to maximize the benefits gained through Rolfing, the practitioner gives instructions and exercises during the sessions which help to retrain the individual in the proper use of her body. These exercises emphasize maintaining the harmony between the body and the laws of gravity. A very important aspect of Rolfing, especially in regard to retaining the benefits gained from the restructuring process, is that of proper body consciousness. The Aston–Patterning movement classes are extremely beneficial in that they give the newly Rolfed person guides as to how to best use her body in everyday situations without falling into the negative movement patterns that had precipitated the need for Rolfing in the first place. For more information on Aston–Patterning, please refer to the section on Aston–Patterning.

For more information contact:

Rolf Institute of Structural Integration
P.O. Box 1868
Boulder, CO 80302

Additional reading:

1. Rolf, Ida P., Ph.D. *What in the World is Rolfing?* Santa Monica: Dennis Landman, 1976.
2. Johnson, Don. *The Protean Body—A Rolfer's View of Human Flexibility.* New York: Harper & Row, 1977.
3. *Rolf, Ida. *Rolfing: The Integration of Human Structures.* New York: Harper & Row, 1977.

The Lomi School

The Lomi School was founded in 1970 by Alyssa Hall, M.A., Robert Hall, M.D., Catherine Heckler, M.A., Richard Heckler, Ph.D., and Vincent and Zelita Regalbuto. The emphasis of the Lomi School is placed on creating a balanced way of being. This total balance can only be obtained by working on the physical, mental and spiritual planes as a whole. The Lomi School, recognizing the interrelatedness of these three elements in each individual, uses a very eclectic approach in its efforts to bring about a positive transformation of the mind, body and spirit.

The core of the actual physical Lomi body work is deep tissue manipulation based on the principles of Structural Integration. This core, however, rests on a framework of developing concentration, one-pointedness, the ability to direct energy from a center, and a special sensitivity to the relationships of the different energy forces inherent in each person. In order to deal effectively with such diverse forces, Lomi practitioners use a wide range of techniques such as Polarity Therapy, Structural Integration, Reflexology, Gestalt and Reichian Therapies, Proskauer breathing exercises, principles of Aikido, as well as yoga and meditation.

In order to facilitate the process of unification or balanced way of being, Lomi work places a great emphasis on client participation. It is work that is being done with you, and *not* to you. Through the use of breath and movement techniques the practitioner is able to achieve deeper manipulations, and the client, aside from being able to maximize the benefits of the deep tissue massage, continually develops his power of concentration or centeredness. Through the role of the active participant the client is forced to remain in contact with himself and must therefore constantly confront the changes that are happening to him. In Lomi work emotional and spiritual growth are just as important as the physical progress. The main technique used by Lomi workers to deal with surfacing emotions is Gestalt therapy;

however, Reichian therapy and bio-energetics are also used. The specific techniques vary as to the practitioner. Yoga and meditation are also used in conjunction with these disciplines in order to better integrate the individual's spiritual awareness with his physical, mental and emotional being. The Lomi School through its open, eclectic nature has developed a flexibility which enables it to treat people in a holistic way in order to bring them into a balanced way of being.

For more information contact:

The Lomi School
475 Molino Ave.
Mill Valley, CA 94941
(415) 388-9906

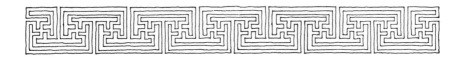

Postural Integration

Postural Integration is the system of body/mind work that has been conceived by Jack Painter, Ph.D. Dr. Painter received his Ph.D. from Emory University in Atlanta in 1961, after which he taught at the University of Miami and did research in the areas of Gestalt and Reichian therapies, psychology and physiophilosophy before developing Postural Integration.

Postural Integration is a special form of body work using the principles of deep connective tissue manipulation in conjunction with Reichian and Gestalt therapies, acupuncture manipulation and movement awareness. The major focus of Postural Integration is the deep tissue manipulation. This technique is very similar to that used in Rolfing, from which it was adapted. The major difference between Rolfing and Postural Integration is that the body work is supplemented with Reichian and Gestalt therapy during each session. In the case of Rolfing this is left up to the discretion of the individual practitioner, many of whom do not use any other techniques in conjunction with their work.

During each session of Postural Integration, Reichian breathing is used to loosen the body and prepare it for the deep connective tissue manipulation that will follow, while Gestalt techniques are used to deal with emotions that surface during the sessions. In the final stages, as the new body begins to come into balance, acupuncture manipulation is used to regulate the yin-yang flow of energy in the body.

Postural Integration, like Rolfing, is not a passive process.

The individual must often move in accordance with the practitioner's movements in order to gain the most benefit from the deep pressure manipulations. Also utilized in Postural Integration is a series of exercises very similar to Aston–Patterning which help the individual to use her body in the most efficient way, maximizing its new flexibility and alignment. Postural Integration usually consists of a series of ten seventy-five minute sessions.

For more information contact:

Jack Painter, Ph.D.
Institute of Postural Integration
1057 Steiner St.
San Francisco, CA 94115
(415) 929-0119

Additional reading:

1. Ebner, Maria. *Connective Tissue Massage, Therapeutic Application.* Edinburgh and London: Churchill-Livingston Press, 1962.
2. Nassberg, Jay, "Postural Integration," (Reprinted from *Issues in Radical Therapy,* Spring 1974)

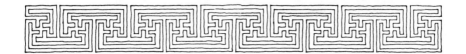

Reichian Therapy

Reichian Therapy, a deep emotional release therapy, is named after Wilhelm Reich, M.D., its founder and pioneer in the field of psychiatry. Before developing his own theories, Dr. Reich was a psychologist working in Vienna as a colleague of Sigmund Freud.

From the very beginning of his work with Freud, Reich was himself an innovator. While still a pupil of Freud, he began to work on a much more direct approach to psychotherapy based on close contact with the patient. At that time the psychiatrist sat behind the couch upon which the patient lay. Reich, however, moved from behind the couch and confronted the patient's resistance directly by pointing out exactly where the patient was consciously or unconsciously holding back some of his feelings.

As Dr. Reich's work continued, he realized that all of the patients who had been cured had achieved a satisfactory sex life while those who had not been cured had not yet attained a fulfilling sex life. From this point Reich went on to formulate his orgastic potency theory which, simplified, is that in order for a patient to be cured he must be able to achieve gratification in the sexual act. Orgastic potency is the capacity for sexual gratification. Orgastic potency is important not only for the full enjoyment of sex, but it also enables the individual to discharge excess energy and thus stabilize himself. This process of discharge and stabilization, which Reich called the orgasm formula, takes place in the following sequence: Tension—Charge—Discharge—Relaxation.

Neuroses in Reichian terms exist only when there is repressed excess energy. Reich believed that the blocking of this bioenergy was due to armoring—the condition that results from energy being bound in a muscular contraction and not being allowed to flow through the body. There are two different categories of armoring—1) natural or temporary and 2) chronic or permanent. The first is necessary and occurs in all living animals when they are threatened. Their bodies tense in preparation for the fight or flight. The second type of armoring is what Reichian Therapy strives to dissolve. This chronic armoring is a result of reacting to ever-present real or imagined inner dangers, such as fear of punishment for crying or fear of punishment for masturbation, rather than a reaction to environmental dangers. This armor then becomes permanent and prevents the individual from feeling deeply in the area of his body where the armor is located. Reich went on to find that, in fact, neurosis is anchored in the armor and that as the armor dissolves in therapy, the orgasm reflex is then released and the body is able to function normally. Along with losing the armor and achieving orgastic potency comes the relaxation of the entire body. It loses its rigidity and the individual is much better able to respond to his daily experiences.

At this point Reich broadened his approach to therapy. He combined direct work on the armored musculature along with psychoanalysis. The results of this new approach (direct work on the body) were excellent, for he found that the body work was a great aid in helping the individual to release his pent-up emotions. This method proved to be both faster and more effective for a greater number of patients than the commonly accepted theories.

This experimentation and research led to Reich's Medical Orgone Therapy. This therapy is based on the principle that the removal of the armor which interferes with the natural flow of energy throughout the body will restore the individual to his proper functioning, and that this method of working directly on the musculature is a more effective way to deal with neuroses than verbal psychoanalysis.

Reich, who had by this time moved to the United States, had a very difficult time gaining acceptance for his theories by the medical community. A large part of Reich's trouble had nothing to do with his medical theories at all, but was of a political nature, for he was an acknowledged communist. In 1954 all of Reich's books were ordered withdrawn from the market and were prohibited from being sold, while any material dealing with orgone energy or orgone accumulators was ordered to be burned. Reich died in 1957 as an outcast in Lewisburg Prison, Pennsylvania. Today, however, there is renewed interest in his very valuable work and it is steadily gaining more and more acceptance.

Reichian Therapy presents a very dynamic and direct way of getting in touch with one's own life energy. This therapy works on two levels—1) the physical or musculature and 2) the verbal or psychoanalytic. The work on the musculature is done through the use of breathing exercises and physical postures which facilitate the muscle spasms that in turn lead to emotional breakthroughs (oftentimes quite dramatic) and the dissolution of the armor. This process of recognizing and releasing the resistances or blocks is carefully watched over by the therapist, who then handles the verbal communication aspect of Reichian Therapy in the way that best suits. Many use Gestalt techniques as well as psychoanalysis.

For more information contact:
The Radix Institute
225 Santa Monica Blvd.
Santa Monica, CA 90401
(213) 395-1555

Additional reading:

1. *Baker, Elsworth F., M.D. *Man in the Trap.* New York: MacMillan, 1967.
2. Bean, Orson. *Me and the Orgone.* New York: St. Martin's Press, 1971.
3. Cattier, Michel. *The Life and Work of Wilhelm Reich.* New York: Avon, 1973.
4. Kelley, Charles R. *Education in Feeling and Purpose.* Santa Monica, CA: Radix Institute, 1974.
5. Lowen, Alexander, M.D. *Physical Dynamics of Character Structure.* Reprinted in paperback as *The Language of the Body,* New York: Grune and Stratton, 1958.
6. Reich, Wilhelm, M.D. *Character Analysis.* New York: Farrar, Straus & Cudahy, 1961.
7. Reich, Wilhelm, M.D. *The Function of the Orgasm* (*The Discovery of the Orgone,* Vol. 1) New York: Farrar, Straus & Cudahy, 1961.
8. Wyckoff, James. *Wilhelm Reich: Life Force Explorer.* Greenwich: Fawcett, 1973.

Bioenergetics

Bioenergetics is a dynamic style of psychotherapy that utilizes physical body work and verbal character analysis to bring about changes in both the personality and in the anatomical structure. Alexander Lowen, M.D., the founder of Bioenergetics, began his training in the field of psychiatry as a student/client and later as a therapist/disciple of Dr. Wilhelm Reich, the originator of Reichian Therapy. Through the process of undergoing and successfully completing Reichian Therapy as a client as well as through his subsequent work as a Reichian Therapist, Lowen gained valuable firsthand knowledge about the body/mind interrelationship. After more than five years work as a Reichian Therapist, Dr. Lowen again felt the desire to enter into therapy as a client. Still convinced of the overall validity of Reich's ideas, but having already completed Reichian Therapy, he began to formulate new approaches and modify certain Reichian techniques that would bring about the results he desired. This process of experimentation on himself was the beginning of Bioenergetics. Over the next twenty years and continuing through today Dr. Lowen has constantly been developing, changing and modifying Bioenergetics as the need has arisen.

"Bioenergetics is the study of the human personality in terms of the energetic process of the body." (4, p. 45) The system of Bioenergetics as stated earlier is strongly rooted in the work of Dr. Wilhelm Reich in that Reich was the first person to emphasize that the body must play a major role in any theory of personality. A major difference between Bioenergetics and Reichian Therapy, however, is that verbal analysis (the discussion and analysis of one's past and present problems and feelings) plays a more important part in the Bioenergetic approach than in the Reichian approach.

Another significant difference between the two therapies is that in Bioenergetics the emphasis is placed on grounding an individual. In order to accomplish this a great deal of work is done on the legs to better facilitate the flow of energy down through the body to the ground. In Reichian Therapy virtually no work is done on the legs and the concept of grounding a person is not used.

The aim of Bioenergetics is to bring about the integration of the mind and the body. This integration will not only enable an individual to understand and feel more comfortable in her body, but it will also make possible a much fuller enjoyment of life in general. Practitioners of Bioenergetics believe that a person's body is the manifestation of how she relates to the world. The healthier and fuller of life energy one's body is, the more vibrant and open one's personality will be. For example, a person in a state of depression doesn't have as much energy to do things or to become involved in even those things which might help to alleviate the depression as does an individual who is functioning normally, because her actual physical energy is lower. Through the dual process of using Bioenergetic exercises to stimulate an increased amount of energy in the physical body, and the discussion of why and how the energy has become cut off or lowered (due to tension or stress and what caused the tension or stress in the first place), a person gains the consciousness and techniques required to be in better control of her life energy. The ability to raise one's physical energy level coupled with the understanding and releasing of the problems that had been constricting the energy brings about change in the personality of the individual.

A cardinal rule in Bioenergetics is that "the body never lies." In the more traditional or strictly verbal schools of psychotherapy (an example of which is Freudian), it is possible for a client to tell the therapist, "No, I am not tense," or "My sex life is fine," when in actuality his neck or abdomen is as hard as a rock indicating the tension that he really feels. In Bioenergetics, as in other forms of body/mind therapy, it is not possible for the client, who may or may not be conscious of how he is truly feeling, to have that kind of an answer accepted by the therapist, simply because the therapist is trained to interpret the body's response, which is a reflection of the truth. Bioenergetic therapists feel that another advantage to the body/mind technique is that it is impossible for a person to completely release his suppressed feelings in a strictly verbal therapy when muscular tension or armoring is holding back those feelings. The client can discuss his feelings forever, but if the feelings remain trapped inside the body, talking will not be able to bring about a long-lasting change until those feelings are released physically. In the body/mind approach an individual is able to release the muscular tension which is holding back the feelings. Once this has occurred he is able to discuss them and realize where they were coming from and why they were there in the first place.

Bioenergetic Therapy, then, consists of two parts: 1) the physical body work or Bioenergetic exercises, in which an individual assumes various postures and does breathing exercises in order to help relieve the muscular tension that is trapping his feelings and life energy, and 2) the verbal analysis which is used to discuss and analyze the person's feelings before or after they have been released. Bioenergetics is a powerful and exciting form of therapy in that the changes brought about in the personality are also reflected in the body structure and vice versa. In short, it is a dynamic style of therapy that strives to bring about positive, long-lasting change by helping people to become aware of and to better understand the body/mind relationship.

For more information contact:

Institute of Bioenergetic Analysis
144 East 36th St.
New York, NY 10016
(212) 532-7742

Center for Energetic Studies
San Francisco, CA
(415) 647-4011

Additional reading:

1. *Keleman, Stanley. *Living Your Dying.* New York and Berkeley: Random House—Bookworks, 1974.
2. Keleman, Stanley. *Bioenergetic Concepts of Grounding.* San Francisco: Lodestar Press, 1970.
3. Keleman, Stanley. *Sexuality, Self and Survival.* San Francisco: Lodestar Press, 1971.
4. *Lowen, Alexander, M.D. *Bioenergetics.* New York: Penguin Books, 1975.

5. Lowen, Alexander, M.D., & Lowen, Leslie. *The Way to Vibrant Health—A Manual of Bioenergetic Exercises.* New York: Harper & Row, 1977.
6. Lowen, Alexander, M.D. *The Betrayal of the Body.* New York: Macmillan-Collier Books, 1969.
7. Lowen, Alexander, M.D. *The Language of the Body.* New York: Macmillan-Collier Books, 1958.

Primal Therapy

Primal Therapy is a radical, deep emotional release approach to therapy that has grown out of the work of Arthur Janov, Ph.D. Dr. Janov practiced insight therapy for seventeen years as a psychologist and psychiatric social worker before developing the primal scream theory. He has been a counselor to several schools for disturbed children and was also on the staff of the Los Angeles Children's Hospital. He now runs The Primal Institute in Los Angeles.

Primal Therapy, like Reichian Therapy, deals with the complete psychobiological functioning of the individual. Both therapies have the same aim—to break down a person's defense system in order to allow her to function normally. The major difference between the two theories is that they approach the same problem from opposite ends. In Reichian Therapy, the major focus is on the biophysical, the de-armoring of the musculature. The breaking down of the physical blocks enables the individual to unlock the repressed emotions that Reich believed were anchored in the armor and caused the formation of the armor in the first place. In Primal Therapy, a more experiential form of therapy, the concentration is centered on first connecting with and then experiencing the "primal pains" (repressed needs and feelings). Once these pains are experienced, they are released through the primal scream, which in turn leads to the individual's ability to release the chronic muscle blocks or armor.

Janov's theory is basically that neuroses develop as a defense mechanism when people realize that they won't be loved for who they are. As children grow and are constantly told not to do this and not to do that, they begin to act in the way that is expected or demanded of them, but which in fact is behaving in a manner that is unreal to themselves. Janov sees the basis for neurosis in this split. As the countless reprimands and negations continue to pile up, the individual finally reaches the understanding that she won't be loved for who she is. This realization which Janov calls the "major primal scene"

94

constitutes the beginning of neurosis—which he defines as "the unreal way people try to be real." From here on neurotic behavior becomes automatic and in many cases people become more unreal than
real. Janov believes that neurosis is actually due to the conflict between the real self and the self that is projected in order to get love.
He feels this conflict is never ending, since the real self has needs
which have not been met. In order to meet these needs the individual
must experience them. Primal Therapy is, as Janov states, a violent
method of attacking and meeting the repressed needs and feelings
that have been building up for years in the unreal self. Primal Therapy uses the force of these repressed years to drive out the trapped
feelings and physical blocks by means of the primal scream.

To qualify for treatment the prospective client has to write an
autobiography, after which she is interviewed and then rejected or
accepted for treatment. If accepted, the individual has to agree to not
smoke, drink, or take tranquilizers. The therapy itself consists of
three weeks of individual counseling during which time the person is
seen for as much time as she needs. This three-week period is usually
followed by a year or so of group therapy.

For the twenty-four hours preceding the first session, the individual is isolated in a hotel room and asked not to leave the room until
her session the next day. The only activity that one is allowed during
this twenty-four hour period is writing. The isolation helps to prepare the person for the primal experience. The first session takes
place in a semi-dark room with the client lying spread-eagled on the
couch to maximize her defenselessness. After discussing her problems, the individual is encouraged to concentrate on a situation that
has aroused a great deal of feeling in her. The first few sessions are
spent getting the individual ready to give up her defense system. As
the sessions progress, she moves closer to having her first primal
scream. It is possible for some people to experience the primal
scream during the first session, while for others it might take a week
or two. When the primal scream finally comes out, it is emitted in
shuddering gasps and body-wracking movements pushed by the
years of repression with which it had been held back. The scream
which is due to reliving the old, painful experience is not a painful
experience in itself. The primal scream is very liberating in that it
causes a dramatic opening in the defense system, enabling the person
to get in touch with the fullness of her feelings. In most cases many
insights are gained through this experience. As the therapy con-

tinues, the primal scream serves both as the cause and the result of the crumbling defense system. Every primal scream strengthens the real self and weakens the unreal self. During the course of the therapy the depth of the primal screams deepen until the balance between the real and the unreal selves is tipped in favor of the real self. Upon reaching the point where the major pains have been both felt and experienced, the unreal self will no longer exist and the client will be normal.

Primal Therapy is a dramatic, forceful approach to therapy. Dr. Janov warns that it is potentially dangerous when practiced by individuals not trained in this specific technique, regardless of their professional background. Primal therapists are trained at The Primal Institute in Los Angeles and only those individuals who have completed this training program are certified by The Primal Institute.

For more information contact:

> The Primal Institute
> 620 N. Almont
> Los Angeles, CA 90032
> (213) 278-2025

Additional reading:

1. *Janov, Arthur, Ph.D. *The Primal Scream.* New York: Dell, 1970.
2. Janov, Arthur, Ph.D. *The Anatomy of Mental Illness.* New York: G. P. Putnam's Sons, 1971.
3. Janov, Arthur, Ph.D. *The Primal Revolution Toward a Real World.* New York: Simon & Schuster, 1972.
4. Janov, Arthur, Ph.D. *The Feeling Child— Preventing Neurosis in Children.* New York: Simon & Schuster, 1973.
5. Janov, Arthur, Ph.D., and Holden, Michael. *Primal Man—The New Consciousness.* New York: Crowell, 1976.

Rebirthing

Rebirthing was founded by Leonard Orr, a young San Franciscan, who had previously worked for est (Erhard Seminar Training). Prior to joining est, he had been a successful salesman and an avid student of spiritual and metaphysical thought. In 1974 he began the Theta Seminars, in which he covered such diverse topics as prosperity consciousness and the concept of physical immortality. Orr came upon his rebirthing therapy theory in the bathtub. He discovered that if he stayed in the bathtub for a long time he would get amazing insights into his infancy. At this point, he began to spend prolonged periods of time in the tub and even started sleeping in it. This started Orr on the journey of unraveling his own birth trauma and led to the creation of the rebirthing process. Rebirth International was founded in 1976.

Rebirthers believe that the birth trauma influences an individual's behavior drastically throughout his entire life unless he can reexperience the birth and thus release its memory. The emphasis in rebirthing is placed on the releasing of these feelings and emotions. All of the techniques employed are designed to facilitate this process. The purpose then is "to remember and re-experience one's birth, to relive physiologically, psychologically and spiritually the moment of one's first breath and to release the trauma of it." (1, p. 69) By freeing oneself of his birth trauma, an individual is thus able to begin to uncover, isolate and identify those areas of consciousness that are unresolved, and begin to work on them.

Orr feels that there are a number of factors which lead to unhappiness. These factors (called the "5 Biggies") are: 1) *the Birth Trauma*; 2) *The Parental Disapproval Syndrome* which is basically that parents take out their hostility towards their parents on their children. The effect of this is that disapproval and negative feelings are handed down from generation to generation. 3) *Specific negatives* are all of the negative attitudes or tapes that one has running about himself such as: No one likes me; I'm fat; I can't make anything work out right; etc. 4) *The unconscious death urge* or the belief that death is inevitable. Rebirthers feel that this unchallenged view of death not only affirms death, but causes many of the illnesses and conditions which lead to death. 5) *Other lifetimes.* These represent to rebirthers an important way of learning about some of one's deep-seated patterns. It is necessary to gain an understanding of these patterns if one is to be able to stop them and gain control of his life.

The rebirthing itself originally took place in a hot tub. "The rebirthee enters the tub with a snorkel and noseplug and floats face down while the rebirther gently holds him in place. The water acts as a powerful stimulus in triggering the experience of being in the womb and being forced out of it." (1, p. 73) This technique is simple and yet quite powerful. After using this method for some time, Orr discovered that it was actually too intense for some people to start in the water, so he developed the dry rebirth. It is now recommended that an individual be dry rebirthed until he has a breathing release. The breathing release is the *most important* aspect of rebirthing. The actual goal of rebirthing is to "merge the inner and outer breath to experience the fullness of divine energy in the body. It is a critical release of all of a person's resistance to life. The breathing release happens when an individual feels safe enough to re-live the moment of his first breath. The breath mechanism is freed and transformed so that from that moment on a person knows when his breathing is inhibited and is able to correct it. This experience breaks the power of the birth trauma over the mind and body." (1, p. 77) Once this stage is reached, a person then goes through the wet rebirths until he has completed the breathing release and frees himself from the negative thoughts and feelings associated with the birth.

Rebirthing is a safe technique that most people find quite pleasurable. Rebirthing can be done in groups, couples or individually, depending upon one's preferences. The number of rebirths required for an individual to complete the breathing release varies from person to person.

Additional reading:

1. Orr, Leonard, and Ray, Sondra. *Rebirthing in the New Age.* Millbrae, CA: Celestial Arts, 1977.

yoga, meditation & the martial arts

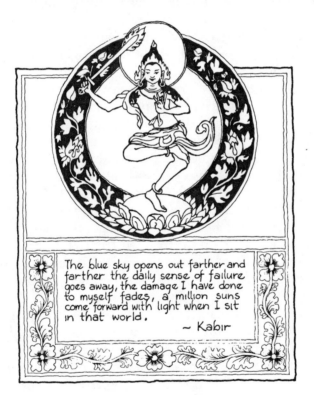

The blue sky opens out farther and farther the daily sense of failure goes away, the damage I have done to myself fades, a million suns come forward with light when I sit in that world.

~ Kabir

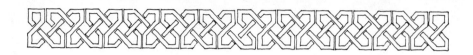

Yoga

The word yoga is derived from the Sanskrit root *yug*, meaning to bind or to yoke. The definition of yoga is the yoking of all the powers of the body, mind and soul to God. One of the six orthodox systems of Indian philosophy, yoga was organized into its present form through the writings of the great saint and yogi Patanjali (500 B.C.). His classic work, *The Yoga Sutras* (also known as *The Sutras of Patanjali),* is comprised of 185 terse and succinct aphorisms that reveal the essence of yogic philogophy. Patanjali named this system Ashtanga Yoga (eight-limbed yoga) due to its having eight stages. The stages are very briefly summarized as "1) Yama (restraints—non-injury, non-lying, non-stealing, non-collecting, moderation in sexual life); 2) Niyama (observances—cleanliness, contentment, austerities, right company and literature, surrender to God)." (2, p. 1)

These first two teachings are the foundation of yoga. If a person doesn't practice them, the following six stages become meaningless. On the other hand, the power gained from perfecting them is so strong that one is able to attain the highest states of consciousness without using any other methods. The next six stages set out practices that help an individual to master the first two. "3) Asana (hatha yoga—a series of 84 main body postures); 4) Pranayama (breath control—8 main techniques for controlling the life force through the breath); 5) Pratyahara (withdrawing the mind from the senses); 6) Dharana (concentration—the development of one-pointedness); 7) Dhayana (meditation that occurs when a person's concentration has become one-pointed); 8) Samadhi (supraconsciousness)." (2, p. 2)

This system of Ashtanga Yoga is the core from which all the other schools of yoga, whether they be called kundalini yoga, hatha yoga, integral yoga or raja yoga (to name just a few), have evolved. In short they are all just variations of the same basic form. Each one stresses a different technique to help an individual to accomplish the same thing—the mastery of the self.

The ancient yogis who lived in the jungles of India developed asanas through their close observations of animals. They noticed that on becoming sick an animal would change its sitting or standing pose and that this would cure the sickness. The yogis discovered that a change in their posture had a very significant effect on the functioning of their glands. This discovery led to the development of hatha yoga. There are some 1,600 asanas, 84 of which are practiced regularly.

Hatha is the form of yoga that is presently so popular in the West. Although primarily thought of as a series of physical exercises (which it is), the real emphasis of hatha yoga lies not in the area of physical fitness, but rather in the development of the subtle body energies. Ha-Tha, which translated means sun/moon, symbolically represents the male and female energies in the human body. "The outgoing male energy and the incoming female energy are controlled by the activities of the right and left energy channels in the subtle body (similar to the ida and pingala nerves in the physical body). The idea of hatha yoga is to withdraw the life force (prana) from the right and left energy channels and take it into the central channel (the shushumna runs up the spine) of the subtle body." (1, p. 48)

This can be accomplished through the practice of asanas (different physical postures) and breathing exercises. When the energy enters into the shushumna it awakens the kundalini (the latent spiritual energy) and forces it to rise up the shushumna. As the energy rises it opens the chakras or subtle body energy centers along the way. The opening of the chakras releases the tension and energy that has been bottled up at these centers. The energy trapped in the chakras is thought to be the cause of all disturbances and disease within the body. Through the constant practice of hatha yoga the energy is able to rise through the chakras up to the crown chakra at the top of the head, producing a state of samadhi or superconsciousness.

There are many different schools of yoga (i.e. Integral Yoga, Iyengar, Ananda Marga, Kundalini Yoga, Okido Yoga, etc.) all of which grew out of the third stage of Ashtanga Yoga (asanas). Each one stresses its own philosophy or attitude towards yoga as well as a certain technique of yoga practice. An example of this type of difference is that in Integral Yoga, as taught by Swami Satchidananda, the emphasis is placed on doing slow, meditative, non-stressful yoga where one doesn't push herself. The breathing is slow, relaxing, and rhythmical. Kundalini Yoga as taught by Yogi Bhajan, on the other hand, is a more forceful form of yoga. He stresses pushing oneself to the limits—"to keep up and be strong." The breathing technique most often used in Kundalini Yoga is the breath of fire, a very deep, hard and fast nostril breath. These two techniques (which create different sensations—one relaxing, one highly energizing) represent different paths to the same goal. An individual interested in beginning yoga or trying a new form can talk to a number of instructors to make sure that she gets involved in the techniques most suited to her personal needs. For more information on yoga classes in your area contact your local YM/YWCA recreation department, community college, community center or natural food store. The *Spiritual Community Guide* is an excellent resource book that lists yoga and meditation classes by location throughout the United States and Canada.

The Light of Yoga Society has a special yoga course for people over sixty. For more information contact:

Light of Yoga Society
2134 Lee Rd.
Cleveland, OH 44118
(216) 371-0078

Additional reading:

1. Dharma Sara Publications. *Between Pleasure and Pain.* Sumas: Dharma Sara, 1976.
2. Hanumann Fellowship. *Hanumann Fellowship Ashtanga Yoga Primer.* Santa Cruz: Hanumann Fellowship, p. 48.
3. *Iyengar, B. K. S. *Light on Yoga.* New York: Schocken Press, 1966.
4. Oki, Masahiro. *Okido Yoga—Healing Yourself Through Yoga.* Tokyo: Japan Publications, 1977.
5. Satchidananda, Swami. *Integral Hatha Yoga.* New York: Holt, Rinehart & Winston, 1970.
6. Vishnudevananda, Swami. *The Complete Illustrated Book of Yoga.* New York: Pocket Books, 1960.

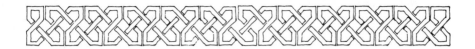

Meditation

Meditation is a discipline in concentration that enables one to unify his consciousness completely. The myriad of meditation techniques taught today all have the same aim—to facilitate the meditator's development of one-pointedness in order that he may then be able to experience the state of transcendental awareness. "Most individuals live on the surface level of consciousness, their grasshopper minds jumping from one subject to another, one desire to another, one distraction to another. But as the mind becomes concentrated in meditation, one learns to extend his conscious control over successively deeper realms of consciousness." (2, p. 2) As a person's meditation deepens his ability to remain focused or one-pointed increases. The state of transcendental awareness is attained when the last thought—the object of the meditation itself—dissolves in the mind. In this completely lucid state of mind, free from all thoughts or disturbances, the meditator is able to experience that "consciousness is always formless and free, and that all the seeming limitations, anxieties and fears are due solely to mental constructions, attachments and desires, born out of the idea that consciousness is limited to the mind and body." (1, p. 55)

The process of calming and centering one's mind is not easy and at times can prove to be quite frustrating. Beginning meditators often notice that their thoughts increase instead of lessen while they are trying to concentrate. This is a normal occurrence. With time and continued practice the mind will settle and become peaceful.

There is a vast array of meditation techniques available today. A few of them will be discussed in greater detail in order to show the great diversity in their approach. In choosing the proper technique for oneself, the most important thing a person can do is pick one that he will practice regularly. As stated earlier, all meditation techniques have the same goal—to help a person develop his concentration.

Any technique will work if the individual has the discipline to meditate regularly.

Mantra Meditation: A mantra is a Sanskrit word that has a known vibratory effect. "Aum," pronounced "Om," is an example of a mantra that is often used in chanting. It is the universal sound of the universe or the all-pervading sound. The mantra (sound energy) is used silently in meditation to create a special psychic state that will further one's meditation. In mantra meditation the meditator (who usually receives the mantra from a teacher) concentrates on repeating the mantra silently over and over again. In many techniques of this kind the mantra is repeated in conjunction with the breath. In all mantra meditation the mantra is to be concentrated upon whenever possible. When the mind drifts away from the mantra, it is to be gently brought back to it.

Transcendental Meditation (TM), the most popular and famous meditation technique in the United States, is a mantra meditation. Brought to the United States by His Holiness Maharishi Mahesh Yogi, transcendental meditation is a simple and effective form of meditation for many busy Westerners. Its appeal lies in the fact that it is completely non-sectarian and has no religious overtones or associations at all. In addition, it is a simple technique to learn and requires that one spend only two twenty-minute periods a day practicing it. Western medical research has attributed many healthy benefits to the practice of TM. It has been proven to be very effective in relieving stress-related conditions, and it seems to improve a person's job performance and his relationships with other people.

The Maharishi has developed a new set of courses called the "Siddhi Preparation" courses for people who have been practicing TM regularly for at least six months. Siddhis are supernormal powers that are attained through a refined mind/body coordination (usually through advanced meditation). In this new program a student will learn to develop such supernormal powers as self-levitation, the ability to see objects normally hidden from view, and super strength.

There are TM centers in every part of the world.

For more information contact:

World Plan Executive   Maharishi International
    Council   University
1015 Gayley Ave.   Fairfield, IN 52556
Los Angeles, CA 90024   (515) 472-5031
(213) 478-3551

Additional reading:*

1. Akins, W. R., & Nurnberg, George. *How to Meditate Without Attending a TM Class.* New York: Crown, 1976.
2. Bloomfield, Harold, et al. *TM—Discovering Inner Energy and Overcoming Stress.* New York: Delacorte, 1975.
3. Dharma Sara Publications. *Between Pleasure and Pain.* Sumas: Dharma Sara, 1976.
4. Easwaran, Eknath. *Mantram Handbook.* Berkeley: Nilgiri, 1977.
5. LeShan, Lawrence. *How to Meditate.* New York: Bantam, 1974.
6. Maharishi Mahesh Yogi. *Transcendental Meditation.* New York: Signet, 1963.

*Shambala Publications, Inc., is an excellent source for books on meditation and spiritual thought.

Shambala Publications, Inc.
  2045 Francisco St.
  Berkeley, CA 94709

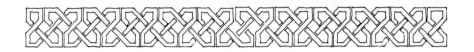

Vipassana Meditation

In the last few years Vipassana (Insight) Meditation has been increasing in popularity in the United States and Canada. Vipassana is a Theravadin Buddhist technique that is based on the Pali Scriptures. Practiced primarily in Burma, Thailand and Ceylon, it is a straightforward (no rituals or ceremonies) approach to meditation that calls for constant awareness. The Vipassana training is one of the most rigorous. The classes are usually ten days long. Each day is filled with ten hours of meditation. The instructors decided on the ten-day retreats because they felt that ten days gives one a good amount of exposure to the range of changes experienced in the meditative process. "From the confusion to being high to more confusion to working through that—so that people get a chance to experience that no one state is it, and that the real teaching is the balance of mind behind the changes. This is the most important teaching." (1, p. 51)

The foundation of the teaching is the concept of *anicca* or impermanence. Everything is transitory—everything is part of the passing show. The Vipassana practice is one of awareness, total awareness or mindfulness of the body, the feelings, the mind, and the objects of the mind—anything that the mind touches. In order to achieve this state of awareness, the meditator concentrates on just one thing at a time. For beginning meditators the technique most often used is that of anapana meditation—the mindfulness of respiration. The meditator focuses her attention on the point of the nostrils where the breath enters and leaves the body. The full breath is not concentrated upon—only the point where it touches the nostrils. After the meditator has developed some familiarity with this process (usually about three days) the attention can then be switched to other objects, such as sensations in one's body. "In the beginning it is as if someone is watching all these objects. The progression of Insight is that when the mind becomes still, mindfulness begins to observe the watcher, to see that actually there is no watcher. There's just watching. That's also a process of arising and passing away— anicca, impermanence. And as it ripens further, the observer and the observed come together. Then there's no difference, just moments of experience with awareness, and there's not that sense of separation and duality. It's just a momentary awareness as part of it, but without a sense of distance." (1, p. 50)

Today the Vipassana teachings are the same as when Buddha first passed them on to his disciples over 2500 years ago. The pureness of the teachings has remained, because the practices have never been written down and left open for interpretation. They have simply been handed down from teacher to student in verbal instruction only. Although 2500 years old, Vipassana is a new method of meditation in the West. U Ba Khin, the great Burmese teacher, was the first person to teach the Vipassana techniques to Western students a little over twenty years ago. Vipassana is an extremely demanding form of meditation. The ten-day retreat is ten days of hard work during which a full range of sensations can be experienced, from incredible pain to indescribable joy. This ten-day training ground is a very powerful and effective method of gaining insight into one's being.

For more information contact:

Insight Meditation Society
Pleasant St.
Barre Center, MA 01005
(617) 355-4373

Additional reading:

1. Fieds, Rick. *New Age Journal,* October 1977, p. 51.
2. *Goldstein, Joseph. *The Experience of Insight—A Natural Unfolding.* Santa Cruz, CA: Unity Press, 1976.
3. Lerner, Eric. *Journey of Insight Meditation—A Personal Experience of the Buddha's Way.* New York: Schocken, 1977.
4. Levine, Stephen. *A Gradual Awakening.* New York: Anchor Press/Doubleday, 1979.

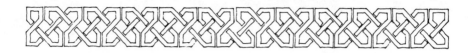

Chaotic Meditation

To many people the term "Chaotic Meditation" seems contradictory. Meditation is most often thought to be quiet, peaceful, sublime and blissful, certainly not chaotic. This, however, is not the case in Bhagwann Shree Rajneesh's technique of Chaotic Meditation. Rajneesh, a brilliant Indian guru, began his career as a professor of philosophy. After a deep study of comparative philosophical and religious systems, he took on his present role as a swami. Using his highly developed intellect, his vast academic knowledge and transcendental wisdom, he has turned a synthesis of Eastern philosophy and Western psychology into a dynamic approach to meditation and spiritual life.

Chaotic Meditation is an interesting and dramatic blending of 1) breath-of-fire yogic breathing, 2) principles of Reichian and Bioenergetic therapies, 3) Sufi chanting and dancing, and 4) more typical meditation practices. The theory underlying Chaotic Meditation is that meditation is a letting go, a surrendering of one's separateness to the wholeness or oneness of the universe. As an individual surrenders more and more of her separateness (which is actually the ego and the attachments to the world) she becomes a clearer channel for the cosmic energy. Chaotic Meditation facilitates this letting go process by forcing an individual to confront her attachments and ego on all levels (physical, emotional, mental, sexual and spiritual). When the ego is dropped a person can then experience the oneness of the universe.

There are a number of different forms of Chaotic Meditation, as Rajneesh is constantly devising new techniques. The basic Chaotic Meditation consists of four ten-minute parts. The first section is devoted to doing the breath-of-fire breathing technique. This is a method of yogic breathing which requires an individual to breathe as deep, hard and fast as possible—through (in and out) the nose only. During this part of the meditation the meditator can stand, sit, walk—do whatever she wants, as long as the breath of fire is continued. A tremendous amount of energy is built up during this section of the meditation. The second stage of the meditation focuses on movement and action. The individual moves with or in the way she feels the energy flowing in her body—dancing, crawling, running, shouting, singing, moaning or jumping. In order to avoid being inhibited when done in a group, individuals often wear blindfolds. The blindfold is also effective in helping one to focus more directly on her inner states. The third part consists of chanting the Sufi word *haun* (pronounced who) over and over again either silently or verbally. The chanting of *haun* is designed to strike the sex energy (kundalini) at the base of the spine. The goal is to excite the kundalini and get it to rise up the shushumna (spinal column of the subtle body) to the top of the head. The chanting is also done in any position that the individual feels comfortable. The fourth and last stage is one of concentration and relaxation. The meditator usually lies on her back and concentrates on the energy flowing throughout her body.

Chaotic Meditation can be done individually or in a group. It seems, however, to be most effective in a group setting, because the group energy heightens one's own energy and experience. As a psychological technique, it is a very powerful method for releasing repressed emotions and physical blocks. As a meditation, it forces a person to surrender her separateness, enabling her to experience the oneness of the universe.

For more information contact:

Ananda Rajneesh Meditation Center
29 East 28th St.
New York, NY 10016
(212) 686-3261

Geetam Rajneesh Sannyas Ashram
P.O. Box 576
Lucerne Valley, CA 92356
(714) 248-6163

Shree Rajneesh Ashram
17 Koregaon Park
Poona 411 011
India

Additional reading:

1. Rajneesh, Bhagwann. *I Am the Gate.* New York: Harper & Row, 1975.
2. Rajneesh, Bhagwann. *The Psychology of the Esoteric.* New York: Harper & Row, 1973.
3. Rajneesh, Bhagwann. *The Mustard Seed.* New York: Harper & Row, 1975.
4. Rajneesh, Bhagwann. *The Book of Secrets.* New York: Harper & Row, 1974.

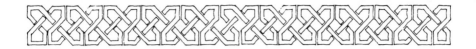

Aikido

Master Ueshibi Morihei (1883-1969) founded Aikido in Japan in 1925. Morihei was a master of many different martial art forms, some dating back to the late 1100s. Having developed the sixth sense (ability to perceive people and their intentions outside of the range of the five senses), it is said that he could throw an opponent without touching him. Aikido is the product of Morihei's lifetime of study of the martial arts, philosophy and religion.

Aikido (*ai*—harmony, *ki*—spirit, and *do*—method) means literally the method of coordinating one's spirit. In Aikido philosophy the spirit rules the body and it is of the utmost importance to unify these two forces. The principles of *ki* and *hara* form the core of Aikido. *Ki* represents the fundamental energy of the universe that connects and relates all things. It is a unifying force that can combine with breath and spirit and become the very emanation of breath and spirit. *Ki* is life itself. Thus, the control of *ki* signifies control over life, health and harmony. The *hara* is the center of *ki* in one's body. It is situated just less than one inch below the navel. In order to gain control of *ki* one must first become centered at his *hara*. This point is one's true center of equilibrium. It is the physical spot where the energies of mind and body meet. Mastery of the *hara*, the heart of the Aikido teachings, is a prerequisite for complete mental and physical coordination.

Aikido is a combination of practical self-defense methods derived from jujitsu, sword fighting, aiki-jutsu, and techniques for the extension of mental energy. It differs from all other martial arts methods in that it is totally defensive. There is no attack in Aikido. The physical training in Aikido is aimed at conditioning a person so that he will be able to respond effectively to an attack. The exercises train a person to free the energy trapped in his tense muscles and to feel the flow of breath and energy throughout his body. Some of the exercises are designed especially to build strength, agility or flexibility, but the overall goal is to bring about the integration of mind and body. Along with the physical exercises, Aikido stresses the use of mental energy, for only by the use of mental extension can an individual truly control his body. Of major importance in Aikido training is the principle of *not* tensing one's body or mind against an attack, but of using them together in a relaxed manner. An example of this is the "unbendable arm" exercise. One student (A) extends his arm while another student (B) attempts to bend A's arm. If A clenches his fist and tenses his arm, B will easily be able to bend it. If, however, A opens his hand, relaxes the arm and concentrates on the energy flowing through the arm and out the fingertips, B will not be able to bend it. The student soon learns the necessity of being able to relax both mind and body in order to blend his *ki* with the opponent's. The Aikido throw is there to flow with and complete the movement of the opponent and not to interrupt it with resistance.

The ethics involved in the practice of Aikido are also different from those in any of the other forms of martial arts. Although Aikido is a totally nonaggressive method of self-defense, a student is taught that he is responsible for not inflicting unnecessary damage on his opponent.

Since Master Morihei's death, Aikido has spread throughout the world and become very popular in the United States, Canada and Europe. A major factor in Aikido's growth is that it is not only an excellent form of self-defense, but it also gives a person a sense of the harmonious quality of the world through the mastery of *ki*.

The study of Aikido as well as any of the other martial arts requires a substantial commitment of time and energy. For more information contact the teachers in your area. A listing of martial arts schools is usually found under Karate in the yellow pages of the telephone book, although classes are frequently available through service or community-sponsored organizations.

Additional reading:

1. Random, Michel. *The Martial Arts.* London: Octopus, 1978.
2. Saito, Morihiro. *Aikido—Its Heart and Appearance.* Tokyo: Japan Publications, 1975.
3. Saito, Morihiro. *Traditional Aikido*—Volumes 1–4. Tokyo: Japan Publications, 1973.

4. Tohei, Koichi. *Aikido in Daily Life.* Tokyo: Japan Publications, 1966.

5. Westbrook, A., and Ratti, O. *Aikido and the Dynamic Sphere.* Rutland, VT: Charles Tuttle Co., 1971.

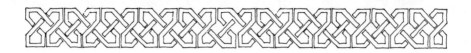

T'ai Chi Ch'uan

T'ai Chi Ch'uan is a system of exercise that dates back to 1000 A.D. Chang Son-Feng, a Chinese philosopher, is credited with developing T'ai Chi after having seen a crane and a snake fight. He noticed during the fight that softness and yielding combined to be very effective forces in a combative situation. He then devised a series of thirteen movements to express these qualities (gentleness and yielding). The basic structure of the thirteen movements was continually expanded upon and refined until the 1800s, when the form emerged as it is known today. T'ai Chi is by far the most popular and best known of the soft forms of martial art.

The aim of T'ai Chi is to help an individual develop her inherent and potential powers. In order to accomplish this, T'ai Chi is designed to greatly increase a person's mind/body coordination enabling her to make better use of her energy. This in turn leads to better health and a state of tranquillity.

T'ai Chi is essentially a technique that employs thirty-nine forms derived from basic movements in nature. For example, one learns to become rooted or grounded like a tree, to breathe deeply and naturally like a large tree swaying in the breeze. The forms are practiced over and over until each movement becomes a part of the next movement and all of the movements flow together, creating one harmonious, whole motion.

In accordance with the Chinese theory of yin and yang (opposite, attracting, balancing energies of the universe), the movement of forms is patterned so that a person always remains balanced. The strong form alternates with the light, the calm with the active, and the expansive with the contractive. Each form requires total concentration and coordination, for every breath, step, movement of eye or hand is regulated and no unnecessary energy is ever to be expended.

The practice of T'ai Chi has become very popular in the United States, Canada and Europe. The reasons for this are numerous.

Aside from being deeply relaxing and energizing, T'ai Chi is well known for its healing powers. The continual relaxed movement in T'ai Chi increases muscle tone and improves circulation. At the same time it opens up the joints, especially the knees, and straightens the spine.

"To truly practice T'ai Chi is to be constantly aware of one's energy, and to cultivate it whenever one has the opportunity to do so." (2, p. 361)

For more information about T'ai Chi contact a martial arts school in your area.

Additional reading:

1. Delza, Sophia. *T'ai Chi Ch'uan: An Ancient Chinese Way of Exercise to Achieve Health and Tranquillity*. New York: Cornerstone, 1961.
2. Berkeley Holistic Health Center. *The Holistic Health Handbook*. Berkeley, CA: And/Or Press, 1978.
3. Huang, Al. *Embrace Tiger, Return to Mountain*. New York: Bantam, 1977.

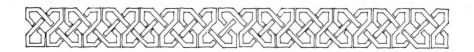

Karate

Karate, meaning "open or empty hand," is a system of exercises first taught by Buddha. It is thought that somewhere in the period of 502–550 B.C. Buddha traveled from India to China. After leading the life of an ascetic for many years, he noticed that his disciples (who were following his ascetic example) were not in good health. In order to remedy the situation he taught them physical exercises combined with breathing exercises. A segment of these teachings became his now famous "Treatise on Limbering Up the Joints" and "Treatise on Limbering Up the Bones." Buddha is also said to have taught at the famous Shaolin monastery, which for centuries served as the center of instruction for over 400 styles of Chinese boxing.

Today there are many different schools of Karate—Chinese, Okinawan, Korean and Japanese. "The techniques depended upon the locality of its study—if the people studying Karate were tall, they specialized in leg techniques; if on the other hand they were short, the specialization was in hand techniques. Thus there are many theories as to the correct movements in Karate." (4, p. 13) While the actual fighting methods differ, the philosophies and theories behind the varying approaches are essentially the same. All schools view Karate as a highly developed art form and not a sport. The Japanese Master Funakoshi Gishin stated that "the essence of Karate is the art of being nonviolent." (2, p. 218) This philosophy is accepted by all of the great teachers and forms a very important part of Karate training.

In all traditions the emphasis is placed on unifying the spirit with the body through intense physical exercises as well as breathing exercises. Karate is a spiritual discipline that aims to bring a student to a state of complete body/mind integration, so that he will be able to perceive the workings of the universe. "The only secret is to practice seriously with perseverance, in order to attain the state of 'mushin' (non-ego) which opens the doors of hara (*the spot where the laws of mind and body converge)** to consciousness. The state of non-ego is the opportunity to be in harmony with nature, to work in accordance with it and to absorb oneself totally in it . . . Karate seeks the unity of body and mind through understanding and assimilating the harmonics of the universe." (2, p. 227)

Although the actual blocks, kicks and punches may differ, most of the major schools of Karate employ the *kata* as their basic mode of teaching. A kata is similar to a classical dance form. Each one consists of a number of offensive and defensive techniques (a minimum of twenty movements) that must be learned in a specific order. In order for a student to progress in rankings he must be able to perform the kata to the teacher's satisfaction. As a student increases in proficiency, the katas to be mastered become longer and more demanding.

Following is a brief explanation of three of the major styles of Karate practiced today:

Shoto-Kan Karate—a Japanese system of Karate developed by Master Funakoshi Gishin in 1922. Shoto-Kan consists of twenty-nine totally different katas. Some are slow and graceful while others are powerful and violent. The perfection of one kata leads to the study of the next, right up to the rank of master. Once a person becomes a master, the true study begins. The Shoto-Kan school has produced the most formidable Karate champions in the recent past.

Goju-Ryu—an Okinawan form of Karate founded by Master Higaonna. The Goju-Ryu method is a combination of *Go* (strength, hardness) and *Ju* (gentleness, softness). The use of synchronized respiration and physical movements characterizes Goju-Ryu. When preparing to block, one's body is soft and the focus is on inhaling. On the attack or while punching and kicking, the individual's body is hard and the concentration is on the exhale.

Tae Kwon Do—a Korean art of self-defense that dates back to 37 B.C. It is a system of exercise designed to harden the body through the practice of various attack and defense forms. Tae Kwon Do is based on the skillful use of punching, jumping, kicking, blocking, dodging and parrying activities. The techniques are essentially linear movements, but a number of circular movements—throws and falling techniques—are also utilized.

---

*Author's insert.

For more information about Karate the yellow pages of the telephone directory usually have a listing of the schools in one's vicinity.

Additional reading:

1. Chun, Richard. *Moo Duk Kwan—Tae Kwon Do: Korean Arts of Self-Defense.* Burbank: Ohara Publications, 1975.
2. *Random, Michel. *The Martial Arts.* London: Octopus, 1978.
3. Toguchi, Seikichi. *Okinawan Goju-Ryu.* Burbank: Ohara Publications, 1976.
4. Ventresca, Peter. *Shoto-Kan Karate—The Ultimate in Self-Defense.* Rutland, VT: Charles Tuttle Co., 1970.

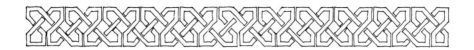

Judo

The Judo that one is familiar with today is the system of Kodokan Judo founded by Professor Jigoro Kano in 1882. Kodokan Judo has its roots in the ancient self-defense methods of jujitsu. Jujitsu, which means "the act of gentleness," developed in the late 1600s as a system of attack and defense techniques primarily used by the samurai. Professor Kano (1860–1938) developed Kodokan Judo by refining the jujitsu methods and by elevating it from an art to a way of being in the world. Professor Kano stressed that Judo, which means "the way of gentleness," was more than an art to be practiced; it was a way of life.

The guiding principle of Judo is to utilize the maximum efficient use of mind and body with a minimum of effort. Applying this concept to combat resulted in Judo's basic premise that in yielding there is strength. The practical effects of this theory can be seen in the following example. "Let us say that the strength of a man standing in front of me is represented by ten units, whereas my strength is represented by seven units. If he pushes me with all his force, I shall certainly be pushed back even if I use all of my strength against him. But if, instead of opposing him, I were to give way to his strength by withdrawing my body just as much as he pushed, taking care to keep my balance, then he would naturally lean forward and thus lose his balance. In this new position he may become so weak, due to his awkward position, as to have his strength represented by only three units instead of the normal ten. I meanwhile, by keeping my balance, retain my full strength of seven units. Now I am momentarily in a superior position and can defeat my opponent by using only half of my strength; that is, half of my seven units or three and one-half against his three. This leaves one half of my strength available for any purpose. Even if I had greater strength than my opponent and could resist him and push him back, it would be wise to give way because by doing so I greatly save my strength while exhausting my opponent's." (2, p. 14)

Of fundamental importance in Judo is an understanding of the laws of movement. According to the theory of Judo, movement is seen as being essentially circular around a point (person) who serves as the center or axis of gravity. In order for an individual to truly act as the center of movement, she must be balanced at hara (the spot approximately one inch below the navel where the laws of the mind and body meet). Judo strives to bring about this welding of the mind and body so that the student will be able to understand not only the laws of movement, but the harmony of the universe as well.

Judo is practiced in two different ways: 1) The *Kata* (similar to the kata method in Karate) is a system of prearranged movements (throws, falls) done in a specific order; 2) *Randori*, meaning "free exercise," is the practice of Judo using whatever moves in whatever sequence one likes as long as she obeys the rules of Judo and does not injure the other person.

The study of Judo is physically and mentally demanding. It requires dedication and a substantial commitment of one's time in order to learn the techniques adequately. However, the rewards (better physical health, increased self-confidence, the ability to defend oneself) of practicing Judo are great.

For more information about Judo in your area contact the martial arts schools listed in the yellow pages of your telephone book.

Additional reading:

1. Goodbody, John. *Judo—How to Become a Champion.* London: William Huscombe, 1974.
2. Risei, Kano. *Illustrated Kodokan Judo.* Tokyo: Kodansha, 1970.

alternative
doctors

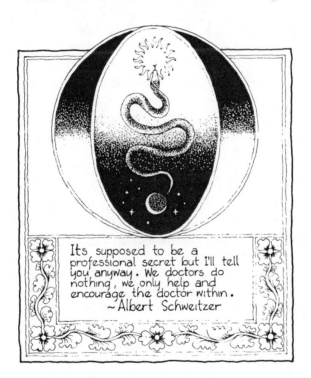

Its supposed to be a
professional secret but I'll tell
you anyway. We doctors do
nothing, we only help and
encourage the doctor within.
~Albert Schweitzer

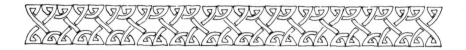

Naturopathy

Naturopathy dates back to the very beginning of the healing arts, when people first began to use the four elements (earth, air, fire and water) in an effort to improve their health. Naturopathic medicine has been defined by Dr. J. E. Cummin as "the science, art and philosophy of adjusting the framework, correcting the mental influences, and supplying the body with its needed elements." Edward Purinton expanded upon this definition when he proclaimed that "Naturopathy is the perfected science of human wholeness, and it includes all agencies, methods, systems, regimes, practices and ideals of natural origin and divine sanction, whereby human health may be restored, enhanced and maintained."

Although the system of naturopathic medicine is ancient, it was first brought to the United States in the late nineteenth century. Naturopathy grew slowly, reaching its height around 1950 at which time the profession experienced a rapid decline in both interest and acceptance. By the end of the sixties, only one accredited college of naturopathic medicine was still in existence and it was hard pressed to continue. The growth of the alternative lifestyle movement has given the naturopathic profession a boost and it is currently experiencing a dramatic resurgence in popularity.

The belief upon which it rests is that "the human body possesses tremendous power to heal itself by means of its mechanisms of homeostasis, which restore balance in structure and function and adapt to environmental changes. . . The naturopathic physician uses only those therapeutic substances and techniques which are in harmony with the body's self-healing processes . . . Ideally, naturopathic methods attempt to stimulate and enhance these natural self-healing powers. Naturopathic medicine is a holistic approach to health; it is medicine for people, not diseases. Each person responds in unique ways to his environment; each has individual strengths, weaknesses and needs. Treating the whole person entails a search for causes at many levels, in the attept to eliminate the fundamental causes of illness, not simply to remove the symptoms." (1, p. 80) The naturopathic approach to healing differs from that of conventional allopathic medicine in that the naturopath is concerned with the relationship between the body, mind and spirit of the individual as well as how he reacts in his environment. Since all of these elements exist or co-exist at all times, the naturopathic theory is that they must all be considered together or holistically, whereas the allopathic physician strives to isolate the symptom analytically in order to identify the disease.

Naturopathy is the only major Western method of natural healing that is not a single branch system of medicine. The techniques practiced by naturopaths span the entire range of natural treatments, massage, psychological counseling, acupuncture, hydrotherapy, botanical medicine, homeopathy and biofeedback, to name just a few. The naturopathic physician is trained to be a teacher as well as a general practitioner, for only through education is it possible to truly practice preventive medicine, which is the aim of the naturopath.

At the present time, only Arizona, Connecticut, the District of Columbia, Florida, Hawaii, Oregon, Washington, Utah, Idaho, Kansas and North Carolina permit naturopaths to practice medicine, although litigation is now pending in a number of other states.

> For information regarding a naturopathic doctor in a specific area contact:
>
> > National Association of Naturopathic
> > Physicians
> > P.O. Box 1648
> > Coeur d'Alene, ID 83814.
>
> The National College of Naturopathic Medicine is currently the only naturopathic school that is recognized for licensing by the state and provincial boards of naturopathic examiners.
>
> For more information contact:
>
> > National College of Naturopathic Medicine
> > 3100 McCormick St.
> > Wichita, KS 67213

Additional reading:

1. Berkeley Holistic Health Center. *The Holistic Health Handbook*. Berkeley, CA: And/Or Press, 1978, p. 80.

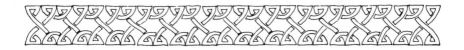

Homeopathy

Homeopathy is a natural system of healing, the underlying principle of which is that a remedy can cure a disease only if it is able to produce symptoms similar to that of the disease in a healthy organism. This concept of using medicine which produces a reaction similar to the disease itself is the direct opposite of the approach taken by conventional medicine, which is founded on the premise of healing with contraries or opposites.

Samuel Hahnemann, a German physician, developed the system of homeopathy in the early 1800s out of his frustration with the inadequacies of the German medical system at that time. Prior to his work with homeopathy Dr. Hahnemann was a very well-known and highly-regarded doctor. Fluent in six languages, he was chosen to standardize the German Pharmacopoeia, and was later elected to the Academy of Science. In 1810 he published a book entitled *Organon of the Art of Healing*, which laid out the basic tenets of a new system of medicine called Homeopathy. Due to his outstanding reputation, he was from the very beginning able to attract other well-known doctors who were also looking for a more effective way to heal the sick. After meeting with some initial bitter opposition, homeopathy quickly spread throughout Europe and is today practiced all over the world.

The basic principles of homeopathy which Hahnemann gave the world in his *Organon of the Art of Healing* are that "medical cure is brought about in accordance with certain laws of healing that are in nature; that nobody can cure outside these laws; that there are no diseases as such, but only diseased individuals; that an illness is always dynamic in nature, and that therefore the remedy too must be in a dynamic state if it is to cure; that the patient needs only one particular remedy for any given stage of his illness, and no other, so that he is not cured unless that remedy is found, but at the best only temporarily relieved." (3, p. 18) These principles along with the homeopathic law "that the rule accepted in conventional allopathic medicine to cure by contraries is entirely wrong and that to the contrary diseases vanish and are cured only by medicines capable of producing a similar affection" (2, p. 46) form the core of the system of homeopathy.

Hahnemann made these discoveries by experimenting on himself with various drugs from the *Materia Medica.* Hahnemann and his colleagues continued this experimentation for six years, during which time they compiled a comprehensive list of poisonings recorded by different doctors in various countries over many centuries throughout the world. Out of this period of experimentation not only was homeopathy born, but also the first Materia Medica that recorded the symptoms which a drug could produce in a healthy person.

At this point Hahnemann's discovery still had one major drawback. The drugs which produced symptoms similar to those of the disease aggravated the symptoms that were produced by the disease. Through more experimentation he learned that by diluting the drug (often to a solution of one part drug to ninety-nine parts distilled water or alcohol) and then submitting it to a hundred vigorous succussions, the mixture would become potentized. He found that not only was the potentized form a more effective healing agent than the straight drug, but it also caused no bad side effects.

The homeopath of today works in much the same manner that Hahnemann and his colleagues did. "By means of exacting study the homeopath learns to pinpoint the specific remedy in the voluminous Materia Medica, which matches one's particular constitution and the stage of the dynamic disease process. Often the remedy that is then prescribed is enough to rectify the imbalance." (1, p. 87)

In the United States the only people legally allowed to practice homeopathy are licensed medical doctors (M.D.'s).

> For information about a homeopathic physician in your area contact:
>
> Homeopathic Information Service of the
> American Institute of Homeopathy
> 910 17th St. N.W., Suite 428-31
> Washington, DC 20006.

Homeopathic Pharmacies:

Humphrey's Medicine Co., Inc.
63 Meadow Rd.
Rutherford, NJ 07070

Luyties Pharmacal Co.
4200 Laclede Ave.
St. Louis, MO 63108

Erhart & Karl, Inc.
17 North Wabash Ave.
Chicago, IL 60602

Additional reading:

1. Berkeley Holistic Health Center. *The Holistic Health Handbook.* Berkeley, CA: And/Or Press, 1978.
2. Hahnemann, Samuel. *Organon of the Art of Healing. The Sixth American Edition.* Philadelphia: Boericke and Tafel, 1917.
3. Vithoulkas, George. *Homeopathy—Medicine of the New Man.* New York: Avon, 1971.

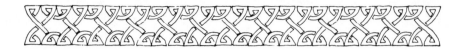

Osteopathy

Osteopathy was founded by Dr. Andrew Taylor Still in the late 1800s. Still (1828–1917) was born in Virginia to missionary parents who raised him throughout the Midwest (at that time the frontier). Although his boyhood adventures on the frontier instilled in him a love of nature, he did not turn first to medicine as a career. In his early life he was very active politically. He served in the Kansas legislature where he espoused controversial causes such as universal suffrage and the end of slavery. In fact, when he began his first Osteopathic College it was open to men and women, black and white. After the Civil War he turned his attention to being a frontier doctor, but was very dissatisfied with the results he was obtaining using the standard medical practices of his time. In the spring of 1864 a spinal meningitis epidemic struck Missouri, killing three of his children. This tragedy pushed Still into beginning his own experimentation in the hopes of alleviating the suffering of humankind. This research led to the science of Osteopathy.

An important factor in the Osteopathic approach to medicine is the fundamental belief in the health or wellness of the body. Dr. Still believed that the body had a predilection for health, and had within it the forces and chemicals necessary for the maintenance of good health. He recognized the healing power of nature and that unless the natural laws of healing were followed a cure was impossible to achieve. An example of this is a broken bone; the doctor sets it, but nature mends it. Dr. Still felt that health was the body's ability to meet various forms of ecological challenge adequately, while disease was the normal response to an abnormal body situation. "We say disease when we should say effect, for disease is the effect of a change in the parts of the physical body. Disease in an abnormal body is just as natural as health when all the parts are in their proper place." (2, p. 20) This outlook formed the underlying difference between his approach and the conventional medical techniques of his time, for he was interested in finding health, while the standard medical doctors were trying to find disease.

The osteopathic system is based upon treating the patient holistically, mind/body and spirit. Osteopaths believe that the body is integrated through the circulatory and nervous systems. Based upon this theory of integration, they feel that an abnormality or disease in one part of the body is more than that, for it has affected the entire body in some way. Keeping in mind this concept of "the unity of the body," the problem can then be diagnosed and treated. The cornerstone of the osteopathic system of healing is the *structure-function principle*. A simplified explanation of this principle is that an abnormality in structure (i.e. displaced vertebra, torn ligament, etc.) causes an abnormality in the physiology of the body. The physiological changes are the result of a breakage in the normal nerve response and blood circulation brought on by the change in the physical structure. Since the structure-function principle is the foundation of their whole profession, osteopaths place great emphasis on the musculoskeletal system which they view as the mirror of disease in the body. Through their techniques of manipulation, they are not only able to cure the structural problem such as dislocated vertebrae, but the coinciding internal (physiological) ones as well. An example of this is stomach ulcers. Stomach ulcers are often known to osteopaths to produce pain in the upper back. By adjusting the upper back the ulcer is many times healed.

Osteopathy today differs very little from standard medicine. The osteopathic physicians, while continuing to employ their manipulative techniques, are now using other therapeutic means including drugs and surgery. In most states osteopaths enjoy the same status as medical doctors.

For more information contact:

American Osteopathic Association
202 East Ohio St.
Chicago, IL 60611

American Osteopathic Association
Farragut Medical Bldg.
Washington, DC 20006

Additional reading:

1. Hoag, J. Marshall. *Osteopathic Medicine.* New York: McGraw-Hill, 1969.
2. Northrup, George. *Osteopathic Medicine.* Chicago: Private Printing, 1966.

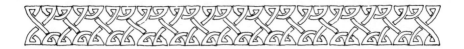

Chiropractic

The Chiropractic system of medicine was discovered in 1895 by Daniel David Palmer in Burlington, Iowa. Palmer (1845–1915) was born in Port Perry, a small town in Canada near Toronto. As a young man he immigrated to the United States, where he worked at a variety of trades including that of grocer and teacher before he became interested in the healing arts. Palmer first studied healing with Paul Caster, the internationally known magnetic healer. He practiced magnetic healing for ten years before he discovered Chiropractic. On September 18, 1895, Harvey Lillard, a deaf man, came to Palmer for treatment. Palmer, curious as to the cause of Lillard's deafness, discovered that it had occurred almost instantaneously seventeen years before, at the same time Lillard felt something give way in his back. Palmer then located a vertebra which appeared out of place in Lillard's back, and reasoned that if it were put back in its proper place Lillard's hearing might return. Using a sharp thrust of his hand Palmer returned the vertebra to its proper position. The results were promising, so he continued treating Lillard for one week, at the end of which Lillard stated he could hear normally, and the science of Chiropractic was founded.

Palmer believed, much as Dr. Still and the osteopaths, that health was the adaptation of the internal environment of the body to the external environment. Disease, he stated, "was not an entity invading the body, but an alteration of body function. Disease is not a thing but a condition—an abnormal performance of certain morphological alterations of the body; agencies and conditions which the body can't adapt to sway the capacity of energy above or below normal, inducing the functional aberration and structural alterations known as disease." (1, p. 11)

Palmer based the Chiropractic system upon the concept of the "innate intelligence" of the body. According to this idea, the inherent wisdom of the body, that which controls the body's vital functions, is transmitted through the nervous system, which he viewed as the system of communication for the entire body.

Chiropractors feel that "disease, whether functional or organic, involves a disturbance of the normal control and communication of the nervous sytem." (1, p. 51) Thus the ability of the body to function in a healthy manner depends on the nerves being free from impingement in order to transmit the needed information effectively.

In order to keep the nervous system free from disturbance, chiropractors focus on the spine (the center of the nervous system). The heart of the Chiropractic philosophy rests in the idea that subluxations (displacements) of the vertebrae of the spine can produce a virtually unlimited array of symptoms which can often be cured by Chiropractic adjustment or manipulation.

Chiropractors are "primarily concerned with maintaining the stability of the self-regulating systems of the body in order to allow the recuperative powers of the body to function normally." (1, p. 80) In the Chiropractic system of healing there is less interest in intervening in the processes of the body, and more emphasis placed in creating the right circumstances which will allow the body to heal itself. Chiropractic physicians use many diagnostic techniques including, but not limited to, X-ray, palpitation, and mobility tests. The focus of their treatment still is the physical adjustment of the body.

The growth of the Chiropractic method of healing since its inception in 1895 is nothing short of phenomenal. It is now practiced all over the world and is continually gaining both support and acceptance for the simple reason that many people have found it has worked for them in cases where standard medicine has not.

For more information contact:

American Chiropractic Association
2200 Grand Ave.
Des Moines, IO 50312

Additional reading material:

1. Dintenfass, Julius, D.C. *Chiropractic—A Modern Way to Health.* New York: Pyramid, 1970.

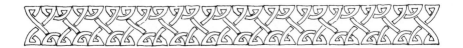

Naprapathy

Naprapathy is the science and art of healing through the manual manipulation of the connective tissue. In 1903 Oakley G. Smith was a young and highly regarded chiropractor. He had served as the Dean of the faculty of the American School of Chiropractics and had developed the Smith System of Spinal Diagnosis. Despite his impressive credentials and the success he had achieved as a chiropractor, Dr. Smith was not satisfied with his profession. In 1904 he traveled to Czechoslovakia in order to observe the practice of *Napravit.* Napravit (which means to correct) is a manipulative healing art practiced in the Slavic countries since the early 1800s. Combining his knowledge of Chiropractic with his research in Napravit, Dr. Smith came to a new conclusion—that derangement in the connective tissue is the primary cause of ill health. This differed from Chiropractic theory in that it is founded on the idea that the main cause of illness lies in bone displacement as in the case of subluxation of the spinal vertebrtae. Dr. Smith returned to the United States and founded the science of Naprapathy in 1905.

Inherent in the philosophy of Naprapathy is the belief that the human body is self-healing and self-regulating, that health is not a stable condition, but a dynamic (ever-fluctuating) process which finds the body continually adapting its internal (biochemical) environment in order to remain in a state of equilibrium with its external environment. The ability of the organism to maintain a state of homeostasis is the Naprapathic definition of good health. Working in accordance with these basic principles, the Naprapathic physician views the body in a holistic manner—"as a whole life source." (1, p. 4)

The Naprapath works in conjunction with nature. His manipulations are aimed at releasing the irritation to the nerves or blood vessels which in turn will restore the body to its proper functioning. "Naprapathy's therapeutic contribution is really the removal or lessening of restraint which is followed by a natural or homeostatic development of health." (1, p. 5)

Naprapathy is the only therapy which claims that soft tissue disease is the primary cause of body disorder. Naprapaths, like Chiropractors, employ hard tissue manipulations as a significant part of their treatments. Chiropractors, however, consider this to be their major curative technique, while Naprapaths see it as merely a tool in the treatment of either stretched or buckled soft, connective tissue. Where Chiropractors are concerned with bone dislocations, Naprapaths believe that disease is caused not so much by the location of an individual vertebra, but rather by "the tension exhibited by the vertebral connective tissues. Stretched connective tissue is indicated by a minimal tension area and buckled connective tissue is indicated by a maximal tension area." (1, p. 5) The Naprapathic and Chiropractic manipulations are also quite different. "Chiropractors use a technique called 'the thrust'—a quick, single and deliberate movement of bone to its assumed normal position. Naprapaths, on the other hand, use a system of directions which are delivered by the hand and are rhythmic, gentle, repetitious and specific." (1, p. 5) In summary, Naprapathy is a system of manually applied movements designed to bring motion, and with it the release of tension to abnormally tense and rigid ligaments and muscles.

> For more information about Naprapathy or a Naprapathic physician in your area contact:
>
> > American Naprapathic Association
> > 9772 South Prospect Ave.
> > Chicago, IL 60043
> >
> > Chicago National College of Naprapathy
> > 3330 North Milwaukee Ave.
> > Chicago, IL 60641
> > (312) 282-2686
>
> Additional reading:
>
> 1. *The Voice of Naprapathy.* Chicago: American Naprapathic Association, Vol. 78, No. 1, p. 5

selected additional topics

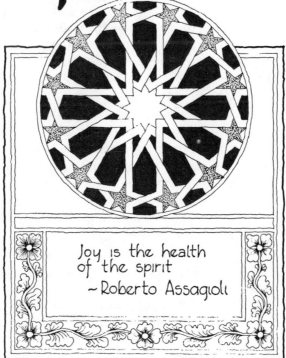

Joy is the health
of the spirit
~ Roberto Assagioli

The Bates Method of Vision Improvement

The Bates Method is a self-healing system of visual reeducation. It is named after Dr. William Bates, the founder and pioneer in the field of retraining the eyes in order to enable them to heal themselves. Dr. Bates, who died in 1931, was a world-renowned ophthalmologist who did his clinical research in the early 1900s at Columbia University and was later associated with Bellevue and Harlem Hospitals and the New York Eye Infirmary.

Dr. Bates believed that focusing is a function of the extrinsic muscles, and not the lens, as the commonly accepted theory postulates. He undertook a wide range of experiments including the surgical removal of the lens as it is done in a cataract operation. Even after this surgery Dr. Bates found refractive error—nearsightedness, farsightedness and astigmatism—problems usually associated with the lens. Furthermore, he was still able to train the eye to see and accommodate at different distances without either the lens or glasses. If the lens then was not the cause of refractive error, what was? He theorized that the psychological aspect of the mind through the brain and nerves controls the actions of the muscles, and that a mind under stress and strain is likely to produce erratic muscle reactions. According to Dr. Bates this includes the reactions of the muscles which control accommodation. He went on to prove clinically many times that most refractive errors are caused by poor coordination be·tween the mind and the eye, and that many of them result from an easily correctable muscle imbalance.

For the last twenty-five years of his life, Dr. Bates dedicated himself to developing a system for improving vision based upon his clinical findings. These were primarily that 1) vision is greatly influenced by mental and emotional stress and strain; 2) vision is clearest when people are relaxed and healthy; 3) stress and strain can be relieved by practicing simple relaxation techniques; 4) the farsight-edness that most people develop in their forties is not inevitable; through the aging process people lose the flexibility of their muscles and thus the eyes are less able to accommodate unless exercises are done to keep these muscles in good condition; 5) nearsightedness and farsightedness are not permanent or hereditary disabilities deter-mined by the fixed shape of the eyeball; 6) that in fact the shape of the eyeball is not fixed—it can and does change constantly in re-sponse to many factors, including tense muscles; 7) if an eyeball does not change shape, it is due to either tense muscles that are holding it rigid or to flaccid muscles that are not able to exert enough force on it; 8) eyeglasses are not beneficial, but are a harmful crutch which perpetuate the errors in the eye and don't help treat the underlying cause of the visual malfunction.

The Bates Method is basically a set of techniques that work to im-prove the mind/eye coordination which has been impaired by strain and tension. Although the Bates Method has been helpful for thou-sands of people, this system has never gained acceptance in the United States. Before his death Dr. Bates challenged the American Medical Association to investigate his theories and prove him wrong. The AMA never did. In Germany, however, the government uses the Bates Method in the public school system and in its armed forces. Probably the single most famous student of Dr. Bates was the philosopher Aldous Huxley, who at the age of sixteen had to read Braille. Even though his vision never returned to 20-20, through the use of this method Huxley was able to read without glasses and without strain. He was so grateful to Dr. Bates that he wrote a book on the subject entitled *The Art of Seeing.*

The core of the Bates Method is a series of simple techniques which can be learned and used with great success from the books listed below. If, however, there is a Bates teacher or a doctor trained in the Bates Method in the area, it is recommended that he or she be consulted. Although only a few of the original Bates teachers are still active, there is a new group of teachers who combine this work with tension reduction techniques and emotional release therapy. These new teachers use the Bates work in conjunction with Gestalt, Bio-energetics, Reichian therapy and natural healing principles in order to unlock the stress that is causing the visual error.

For more information contact:

Koen Kallop
Northern California School of Massage
    and Natural Therapeutics
116 Elm St.
San Mateo, CA 94401
(415) 348-1034

Dr. Charles Kelley
The Radix Institute
225 Santa Monica Blvd.
Santa Monica, CA 90403

Gestalt Center for Psychotherapy &
    Training
150 East 52nd St.
New York, NY 10022
(212) 752-1932

Additional reading:

1. *Bates, William, M.D. *The Bates Method for Better Eyesight Without Glasses*. New York: Pyramid Books, 1973 (fourteenth printing).
2. Benjamin, Harry. *Better Sight Without Glasses*. London: Health for All Publishing Co., 1958.
3. Corbett, Margaret D. *How to Improve Your Eyes*. Los Angeles: Willing Publishing, 1938.
4. Huxley, Aldous. *The Art of Seeing*. Seattle: Montana Books, 1975.
5. Jackson, Jim. *Seeing Yourself See*. New York: Saturday Review Press & E. P. Dutton, 1975.
6. Kelley, Charles R. *New Techniques of Vision Improvement*. Santa Monica, CA: Interscience Workshop, 1971.
7. Peppard, Harold, M.D. *Sight Without Glasses*. New York: Signet Key, 1956.
8. Rosanes-Berret, Marilyn, Ph.D. *Do You Really Need Eyeglasses?* New York: Hart, 1974.
Phonographic Record—*Improve Your Eyes Without Glasses*. Jim Wolfe, Wolfe Records, Seattle, 1977.

Sensory Awareness

Sensory awareness is a discipline of attention to what's real, moment by moment—breath, movement, light, sound, temperature. It is constant and total attention to the reality of one's unfolding experience. The term "sensory awareness," which has recently been loosely applied to many techniques in the human potential movement, was first used by Charlotte Selver in 1950 as a name for the work that she had learned from Elsa Gindler. Gindler was a physical education teacher in Berlin, Germany, when she was stricken with tuberculosis. In 1910 the medical profession could not offer much hope for people stricken with TB. After receiving no help from her doctors, Gindler decided that if she could be patient enough to listen to her body, she ought to be able to sense her own inner processes and thus discover methods that she could use to facilitate her healing. Within a year Gindler had healed herself. She spent the remainder of her life (until 1961) teaching people to learn how to sense their own functioning. Charlotte Selver was one of the first people to bring Gindler's teachings to the United States. Since 1938 Selver has been actively and constantly developing and refining her approach to the Gindler work. The name "sensory awareness" was chosen to single out the awareness of direct perception from the awareness of the intellect.

Sensory awareness is based on the idea that in human beings there is a division between the intellectual process and the process of sensory awareness. Simply put, the division is between what one perceives and what one thinks about what she perceives. The dominance of the intellect and the abstract thoughts and language from which all of one's ideas arise have made the civilized world possible. In the process, however, it has robbed an individual of the opportunity to truly know her own experiences and has thus resulted in an alienation of the individual not only from nature, but also from herself. "The so-called mind/body split refers to the immense and still growing separation in our culture between the intellectual processes and sensory experience. No one can doubt that this is a catastrophic fact. On the one hand we have the abstract information as well as the theories, cliches, stereotypes, and fantasies that are the stock in trade of most people's conversation, reading, writing, and trains of thought—in a word, of their consciousness. On the other hand is experience, which for a great many people today is practically limited to comfort and discomfort." (1, p. 8)

The goal of sensory awareness is to enable a person to get in touch with her true experience. The true experience is real only when it is perceived directly—either through bypassing or short-circuiting one's intellectual perception. In order to bring about the desired change in awareness from intellectual understanding to direct perception, the sensory awareness techniques apply meditative attention to the performance of the everyday functions of living. Through simple experiments involving activities such as sitting, moving, breathing and touching, one begins to explore one's nature in its fullness.

For more information contact:

Charlotte Selver Foundation 32 Cedars Rd. Caldwell, NJ 07006	Charlotte Selver and Charles Brooks Green Gulch Farm Star Route Sausalito, CA 94965

Additional reading:

1. Brooks, Charles. *Sensory Awareness—The Rediscovery of Experiencing.* New York: Viking Press, 1974.

Breath Awareness

Proper breathing plays a vital role in improving one's psychological, physical and spiritual well-being. For centuries Eastern mystics and yogis have recognized the breath as being an extremely valuable tool for increasing one's awareness. The fourth stage of Yoga (prana-yama) is devoted to gaining control of one's breath. Through the practice of various exercises, an individual learns to not only control his breathing, but also to restrain and quiet the flow of life force energy (prana). According to yogic philosophy, there is a direct relationship between life force activity and the rate of breathing. "When the life force is operating smoothly the breath is calm and regular, but when it is excited, breathing becomes erratic. Breath control is designed to still the mind and achieve transcendental awareness by controlling the life force. This is done by regulating and harmonizing the breath in particular patterns." (1, p.51)

The breath is a unique bodily function in that it is the only one which can be either controlled or automatic. Throughout most of a person's life he, without thinking about it, automatically breathes. At the same time, however, an individual is capable of consciously changing, at will, his breathing pattern by, for example, taking a deep breath. The breath, therefore, serves as a bridge between the conscious (central) nervous system and the unconscious (automatic) nervous system. Through observation one is able to ascertain where his breath is (chest, abdomen) and how he is feeling. Once this has been determined, the breath can then be used as a tool, for by changing one's breathing, a person is able to change his energy or mood.

The easiest and most important method for attaining and maintaining good breathing is regular exercise. There are also a number of Western therapeutic techniques concerned with the important role that proper breathing plays in an individual's physical, emotional and psychological health. Reichian therapy and Bioenergetics both focus on helping a person to develop full movement of breath

141

throughout his body. In order to accomplish this, they strive to break down the physical armoring (muscular tension) which blocks the flow of energy and then re-pattern the person's breathing to facilitate the maximum flow of energy in the body. (For more information on Reichian and Bioenergetic therapies, check the Reichian and Bioenergetic chapters.)

Another very effective, though different, method of breathing is taught by Magdalene Proskauer in her Breath Awareness classes. Ms. Proskauer, a trained physical therapist from the University of Munich, has been helping people with breathing difficulties (asthma, tuberculosis) as well as normally healthy people to better regulate their own breathing since the 1920s. Her approach differs from the others in that she does not employ controlled breathing patterns. The aim of her work is to enable a person to relax and breathe in his own way in order to experience his natural rhythm. Through these exercises which are slow and gentle an individual is able to relax deeply and release stored-up tension. Ms. Proskauer teaches these exercises in a weekly one-hour class at her home in San Francisco.

Additional reading:

1. Berkeley Holistic Health Center. *The Holistic Health Handbook.* Berkeley, CA: And/Or Press, 1978.
2. Dharma Sara Publications. *Between Pleasure and Pain.* Sumas: Dharma Sara, 1976.
3. Geba, Bruno. *Breathe Away Your Tension.* New York: Random House—Bookworks, 1973.
4. Rush, Anne. *Getting Clear—Body Work for Women.* New York: Random House—Bookworks, 1973.

Isolation Tank Technique

The Isolation Tank Technique is the development of Dr. John Lilly. A graduate of the California Institute of Technology and the University of Pennsylvania Medical School, Lilly is a prolific writer (author of eight books) and researcher in a wide range of medically related fields including biophysics, neurophysiology, electronics, and neuroanatomy. Although probably best known for his research in the area of human/dolphin relationships, he is also a qualified psychoanalyst, and is commonly regarded as one of the pioneers of the humanistic psychology movement. Dr. Lilly has been studying the effects of isolation ever since he first developed the isolation tank in 1954 at the National Institute for Mental Health.

The isolation tank grew out of Dr. Lilly's study of the workings of the mind. The reasoning behind the tank was based on one of the tenets of scientific experimentation, "in order to adequately study a system, all known influences to and from that system must either be attenuated below threshold for excitation, reliably accounted for, or eliminated to avoid unplanned disturbances of that system. Disturbances from unknown sources may then be found and dealt with more accurately." With this concept in mind he devised the isolation tank, a method which would enable him to study his own mind and its processes free from outside stimulation. In the twenty-five years since its inception, Lilly has spent not only hundreds of hours in the tank, but has been continually working at refining the tank itself. Since 1973 he has worked with many men and women who have volunteered to try the tank and record their experiences. These experiences are told in his book *The Deep Self*.

The isolation tank is built to cut out as much external stimulus as is possible. It is kept totally dark inside, almost all noise is blocked out, and the gravitational effect on the body is neutralized due to a saturated solution of Epsom salts and water. At the solution of 1.30 grams per cubic centimeter, a person is able to float freely in a supine position and have her whole body at or near the surface of the water. The temperature in the tank is set between 93°–94° Fahrenheit and is held constant within one-tenth of one degree. This almost total isolation is designed to "free the body from the necessities of external reality by cutting physical input patterns," (1, p. 31) down to the lowest level possible.

The effects of the isolation tank are manifold and differ from individual to individual. The tank can be used solely as a method for personal relaxation; it can also be used as a tool for tremendous psychological growth. The cessation of external input and the forces of gravity that one experiences inside the tank enables an individual to attain the deepest state of rest within an extremely short period of time. A special float has been developed that enables people to sleep in the tank without fear of their head turning sideways. Due to the deepness of the state of relaxation produced, a short nap in the tank is oftentimes equivalent to a whole night's sleep in a bed. The tank is a valuable instrument for psychological growth in that it "assists a person in expanding the awareness of his internal state of being. This augmented sensitivity to the ranges and varieties of the inner world enriches not only that realm, but of course the everyday world where one does most of his living. The tank experience is useful in isolating the variables, in finding who is doing what to whom, that who and whom are the same person—one self. In the tank there is nothing happening, but what you are doing or aren't doing."

At this time there are few isolation tanks available for general public use. Dr. Lilly has worked with Glen Perry of the Samadhi Tank Company in designing and building portable isolation tanks for use in one's own home.

For more information contact:

Samadhi Tank Company
2123 Lakeshore Ave.
Los Angeles, CA 90039

Additional reading:

1. *Lilly, John. *The Deep Self.* New York: Simon & Schuster, 1977.
2. Lilly, John. *The Center of the Cyclone.* New York: Julian Press, 1972.
3. Lilly, John. *Simulations of God.* New York: Simon & Schuster, 1975.

Gravity Guidance

The Gravity Guidance System of exercise is the result of twenty-eight years of research by R. Manatt Martin, M.D., D.O., D.C. Dr. Martin's methods of physical fitness enable individuals to not only live more harmoniously with the effects of gravity, but to actually utilize gravity as a tool working for their benefit. After being faced with numerous cases of back pain, Dr. Martin began to draw on his past experience as a gymnast in order to devise a system of exercise which would help alleviate the downward pull and accompanying pain of the force of gravity. He soon found that his series of exercises were working far better than the medication and surgery that he had previously been prescribing.

The statistics concerning back problems are absolutely mind boggling. "Every day over 8,500,000 Americans are in bed with a backache, and with each passing year, this astronomical figure multiplies. Eighty-three percent of the world's inhabitants will suffer from a disabling backache sometime in their lives." (1, p. 1) Until recently the overwhelming consensus of medical practitioners has been that the primary cause of backache is due to the effect of gravity on the erect human posture. The stress from the force of gravity resting along the vertical spinal column rather than upon a horizontal spinal beam, as in other land animals, makes it exceedingly difficult for an individual to maintain proper posture and a strong back. Dr. Martin, however, does not believe that the problem of backache is due to the process of evolution; in fact, he believes that "an individual's ability to change his postural relationship with respect to gravity, which the vertical spinal column allows, is one of the great human attributes." (1, p. 4) The ability to practice a virtually unlimited number of postures affords the human body the chance to experience the full range of the gravitational force from compression, when the body is erect, to decompression and elongation, when the body is inverted. This gives a person the opportunity to control the environmental stress of gravity on her body in a way that is not possible for other animals. Dr. Martin's theories are not new; they can be traced back to hatha yoga, an ancient system of healing, based upon a set of physical body postures or asanas. Through the continued practice of these asanas a person experiences the full range of gravitational force on her body. Yoga has been found to increase suppleness, longevity and general health.

Practitioners of the Gravity Guidance System believe that the most effective tool for the prevention and cure of backache is "properly planned and guided postural change." (1, p. 8) By changing the position of one's body, an individual is able to work with the force of gravity and use it as a "stress equalizer allowing it to become an adjuster of the body's tissues and structure by creating equilibrium through a combination of positions." (1, p. 30)

When a person assumes an ordinary posture (standing, sitting, lying) the force of gravity compresses the body by constantly pressing down on it. To somewhat offset this continual downward force, it is important for the individual to learn some new postures which will decompress or elongate her body, such as hanging upside down. Dr. Martin has divided his system into two sets, each with three categories of postures. The first set, the *common postures,* are used in the everyday situations of work, play and sleep. These positions give rise to the compression of the body due to the force of gravity upon it. This set is comprised of "the erect posture—sitting or standing, the horizontal posture—lying down, and the flexed posture—bending forward." (1, p. 32) The second set is that of the *uncommon postures* which are employed to counter the effects of gravity by helping to decompress and elongate the body structure. This group is made up of "the extended posture—bending backwards, the brachiated posture—hanging by the limbs, either the upper or lower, and the inverted posture—standing on either the hands or forearms or hanging by the lower limbs." (1, p. 32)

In order to maintain a healthy, well-toned body it is necessary to use the uncommon postures to help counter the damaging effects of the force of gravity that occur when the common postures are used exclusively. Understanding this need to use all of the postures daily and to help maximize their benefits, Dr. Martin invented exercise equipment which enables everyone to fully use all of these postures. The equipment, "The Gravity Guidance Machine," makes it very simple for anyone to hang upside down, to do deep bends and to hang by their arms as well as to do many other exercises. Along with the equipment Dr. Martin has written the *Gravity Guiding Manual* which shows in detail the various exercises to be done with the equipment. The manual also explains in depth the benefits gained from each exercise. The equipment may be purchased and set up in one's own home. It is not inexpensive, but it is very cheap both financially and emotionally compared to having a bad back or back surgery. The other possibility is to go to one of the Gravity Guidance Centers, where there are trained instructors who help people go through the program for a small fee. Either way it is highly recommended that an individual consult her health counselor before beginning the program.

The Gravity Guidance System, aside from being a very valuable alternative to back braces and surgery, is also an excellent program of exercises which not only help prevent back problems, but are quite effective for maintaining good muscle tone and conditioning for the entire body.

For more information contact:

R. Manatt Martin, M.D.
816 Union St.
Pasadena, CA 91101
(213) 791-1694

Additional reading:

1. *Martin, R. Manatt. *Cum Gravity Living With Gravity*. San Marino, CA: Essential Publishing Co., 1975.

New Games

"Play hard, play fair, nobody hurt" is the motto of the New Games. Stewart Brand, founder and editor of the Whole Earth Catalog and the Co-Evolution Journal, is the single person most responsible for the development of the New Game philosophy. In 1966 Brand was asked by the War Resisters League at San Francisco State College to stage a public event for them. For this meeting Brand invented a number of games which would involve intense interaction between the players and create a lot of opportunities to express aggression. In one of the games (earthball) a big (6 feet in diameter) ball is pushed back and forth on a large field by two teams until one team finally scores. That afternoon there was plenty of competition, but as soon as one team got close to scoring, players from that team would defect and help the other team to stop the goal from being scored. "The players had been competing, but not to win. Their unspoken and accepted agreement had been to play, as long and hard as possible." (1, p. 9) This, in effect, was the beginning of the New Games.

Brand, along with his friend and fellow author, George Leonard, began to investigate games in a new way—from a creative standpoint rather than a competitive one. Leonard was especially interested in the idea of creative play,". . . the experience of a player placed in an open environment and encouraged to use his imagination to devise new play forms. Leonard wrote, 'sports represent a key joint in any society. How we play the game may turn out to be more important than we imagine, for it signifies nothing less than our way of being in the world.'" (1, p. 10)

The first New Games tournament was held in October, 1973, in the Gerbode Preserve, a 2200-acre valley just north of the Golden Gate Bridge. "The chance to participate not only by playing, but by actually making up new games attracted 6,000 people, all of whom actively played." (1, p. 11) This auspicious event launched the New Games concept. The second New Games tournament received national news coverage, and before long the games were being played throughout the United States as well as in England and Australia. In short, the games caught on wherever they were tried. The beauty of them lies in the fact that not only does everyone get a chance to play, but everyone is actively encouraged to play, no matter what age, shape, sex or size. Another important factor behind the New Games' success is that virtually no equipment is needed for most of the games and the equipment needed for the rest of them can be easily made at very little cost.

A New Games Foundation has been established to organize workshops and trainings for tournaments. It also publishes a newsletter which covers the best New Games, new equipment and other pertinent New Games information.

For more information contact:

New Games Foundation
P.O. Box 7901
San Francisco, CA 94120
(415) 664-6900

Additional reading:

1. *Fluegelman, Andrew. *The New Games Book.* New York: Doubleday, 1976.

    (An excellent book which tells everything one needs to know to organize a New Games tournament including instructions for some of the most popular games.)
2. Leonard, George. *The Ultimate Athlete.* New York: Avon, 1974.
3. Orlick, Terry. *The Cooperative Sports and Games Book.* New York: Pantheon, 1978.

A Course in Miracles

A very unusual and effective approach to improving one's ability to experience love is *A Course in Miracles*. The course was developed by two psychologists who prefer to remain anonymous, in the belief that the work should not only stand on its own but that it should not become the basis for another organization, school or cult. The sole intention of the course is to enable people to contact their "natural inheritance"—love. The course came into being through psychic transmissions to one of the psychologists. The other psychologist then typed the psychic information and helped to arrange it in its present form. This process, which continued for six years, produced a textbook, a workbook and a teacher's manual.

The course, which is designed to be self-teaching, emphasizes experience rather than theory. The text presents the foundation for understanding miracles. The theoretical and philosophical aspects of the course are built around the guiding principle that "Miracles occur naturally as expressions of love. The real miracle is the love that inspires them. In this sense everything that comes from love is a miracle." (1, p. 1) The workbook, on the other hand, is comprised of 365 simple lessons or exercises (one for each day of the year) that were developed to enable the student to experience the teachings in the textbook. The course does not have to be completed in one year. An individual is encouraged to work through the course at whatever speed he feels most comfortable; however, it is advised that only one lesson per day be attempted. Aside from this advice, the only other instruction for the course is: "Some of the ideas the workbook presents you will find hard to believe, and others may seem to be quite startling. This does not matter. You are merely asked to apply the ideas as you are directed to do. You are not asked to judge them at all. You are asked only to use them. It is their use that will give them meaning to you, and will show you that they are true.

"Remember only this: You need not believe the ideas, you need not accept them, and you need not even welcome them. Some of them you may actively resist. None of this will matter, or decrease their efficacy. But do not allow yourself to make exceptions in applying the ideas the workbook contains, and whatever your reactions to the ideas may be, use them. Nothing more than that is required." (1, p. 2)

According to the teachings in the course, there are two distinct realms: 1) the real world, the world of knowledge, truth, and the laws of love; 2) the unreal world, the world of perception, time and change. Most people live in a world of perception that they have created by projecting their own internal feelings outward. In other words, if an individual is depressed, he projects those feelings out to the world at large and thus perceives a depressing world. The goal of the course is to help a person give up the world of his individual perception and enter into the world of universal knowledge or love. The workbook, the experiential part of the course, has been divided into two major sections. In the first section the student is assisted in unlearning his old ways of viewing the world. In the second section the student learns how to gain "true perception" in accordance with the universal laws of love. In short, the exercises have been systematically developed to train an individual's mind to a "different perception of everyone and everything in the world." (1, p. 1) An example of the exercises taught is: "Nothing I see in this room [on this street, from this window, in this place] means anything." (1, p. 3) In this lesson the student is to practice applying this idea to whatever he sees (this book does not mean anything; this table does not mean anything, etc.). The lesson should be done no more than twice a day, for no more than a minute at a time.

A Course in Miracles is a unique approach to helping an individual understand the guiding laws of the universe. Through the process of changing his perception about the world, the student is thus able to be a source of love. The end result is a happier, healthier view of oneself and the world in general.

The only way to get the course is to order it from the publisher. The three-volume hardbound set is sold for $25.00 plus $2.00 postage. Due to the interest of many people who have taken, or are taking, the course, study groups and workshops are in the process of being formed by students of the course who are functioning independently of it.

For information contact:

> Foundation for Inner Peace
> P.O. Box 635
> Tiburon, CA 94920

1. *A Course in Miracles.* New York: Foundation for Inner Peace, 1975.

Biorhythm

The study of Biorhythm is the attempt to understand how three internal biological rhythms influence people's lives. The discovery of Biorhythm took place in the 1890s. Dr. Hermann Swoboda, a professor of psychology at the University of Vienna, and Dr. Wilhelm Fliess, a prominent nose and throat specialist in Berlin, first discovered Biorhythm at approximately the same time while doing totally independent research. Dr. Swoboda was initially interested in Biorhythm in conjunction with his research into the theory that there are seemingly rhythmic changes to an individual's mental states. Through analyzing and keeping records of his own patients, Dr. Swoboda discovered that all physical ailments, whether fevers, heart attacks or asthma, would recur in accordance with a 23-day or 28-day cycle and by being aware of and using these cycles one had the ability to predict their recurrence. Dr. Swoboda later wrote a number of highly acclaimed and popular books on Biorhythm.

At the same time, though unaware of his colleague's work, Dr. Fliess, a close friend of Sigmund Freud, had become convinced through his own research that "the best explanation of the ebb and flow of resistance to disease lay in the 23-day and 28-day cycles that are the foundation of biorhythm." (1, p. 44) Dr. Fliess published four books on Biorhythm before his death in 1928, but received little acclaim in his lifetime, for he wasn't able to communicate his discoveries in a clear and concise manner. The third Biorhythm was discovered by Dr. Alfred Teltscher, a professor of engineering in Austria. Dr. Teltscher, influenced by the excitement that Biorhythm theory was beginning to cause, was anxious to see if any rhythms were apparent in the intellectual performance of his students. Dr. Teltscher had noticed previously that even his best students had bad days and their ability to perform at a high level was not stable. After collecting and statistically analyzing his information he discovered that there was a very regular, constantly repeating, internal intellectual cycle of 33 days. During each 33-day cycle a student's mental abilities would vary according to what phase of the cycle she happened to be in at that time. These three cycles (the physical 23-day cycle, the emotional 28-day cycle and the intellectual 33-day cycle) form the basis of the Biorhythm theory.

Biorhythm theory essentially states that everyone from the moment of birth until death is influenced by these three internal cycles. The physical cycle affects a wide range of bodily functions including coordination, strength, and the body's ability to resist disease. The emotional cycle controls mental health, one's moods, perception and creativity. The intellectual cycle is responsible for regulating such things as memory, awareness, and comprehension as well as the logical functions of the mind.

At the time of birth each cycle starts at a neutral or zero point. From this point it continues to rise in a positive phase for half of the length of its complete cycle. The positive phase lasts for eleven and a half days in the physical cycle, fourteen days in the emotional cycle and sixteen and a half days in the intellectual cycle. During the positive phase the attributes, abilities and energies associated with each cycle are high. At the midway point, the cycles change and enter into the negative phase. During the negative phase, the body functions at a lower level while it recharges itself for the next positive phase. When the zero point is crossed the negative phase ends and the whole process starts again.

Due to the fact that the three cycles are of different durations they very rarely all coincide; therefore people are usually influenced by mixed rhythms—some of the cycles will be in a positive phase while another might be in a negative phase and vice versa. The result of this is that our behavior—"from physical endurance to creativity to performance on academic examinations is a composite of these differing rhythms." (1, p. 15) The crucial periods, according to Biorhythm theory, are not when the cycles are in a negative phase, but when they are crossing over from positive to negative or from negative to positive. These days are called the *critical* days. Examples of this are that on physically critical days people are most likely to have accidents and get sick. During emotionally critical times people are prone to fight and become depressed. When one is having an intellectually critical day (her intellectual cycle is switching phases from either negative to positive or from positive to negative) she will experience more difficulty than usual in using good judgment, being attentive and making decisions.

Understanding one's critical days may be the single most important aspect of Biorhythm, because as seen in many scientific and industrial studies, especially in the transportation industry, it can be a matter of life and death. It has been shown through these studies that approximately 56 percent of the single-car accidents that take place occur when the driver is having a critical day. This is quite a high percentage considering one has a critical day only 20 percent of her life. The concept behind Biorhythm is that by becoming aware of and knowing in what phase of one's cycle one is, an individual will not only be able to take precautions on her critical days, but will also be able to maximize her potential by using her abilities at the proper time to bring about the best results. A simple example of this is that it would be unwise for someone to undertake a new and strenuous project when all of her cycles are in the negative phase. Another important example is in medical cases where surgery is necessary. It would make good sense to arrange to have the surgery performed when one's physical and emotional cycles are at high points.

Biorhythm is currently used to the greatest degree by the Japanese and the Swiss, although it is quickly becoming more accepted by a large number of individuals and industries in the United States. At the present time more research needs to be done to determine exactly why Biorhythms work and how they affect people's lives. However, even at this stage in its development, Biorhythm can be an extremely valuable aid as it not only allows an individual to better understand how she is functioning in the present, but it also gives her a means by which she can predict the future, and then plan for it.

Additional reading:

1. Gittelson, Bernard. *Biorhythm/A Personal Science.* New York: Warner Books, 1975.

"Birth Without Violence"

All of the aforementioned techniques are designed to help an individual to heal himself; to aid a person in discovering the wholeness of his being; to allow one to experience the full potential of life. If it is true, as many great healers have postulated, that the birth trauma is the single major cause of an individual's emotional and psychological problems, then this last technique may well be the most important, for its goal is to make the birth experience as gentle, loving and untraumatic as possible. If it succeeds to the degree that many people claim it does, then it might be possible to alleviate many of one's problems before they begin.

"Birth Without Violence" is a system of natural child delivery devised by Dr. Frederick Leboyer, a French obstetrician. Since 1953 Dr. Leboyer has delivered over 10,000 babies. In the course of his work he became dissatisfied with the standard medical procedures for child delivery, which he felt did not realistically take into account the feelings of the newborn baby. This led Dr. Leboyer to develop new obstetrical methods that were oriented towards receiving the new baby in a gentle, warm, loving atmosphere as opposed to the cold and harshly sterile hospital delivery rooms. Out of this experimentation evolved the "Birth Without Violence" child delivery concept.

With the baby's psychological and emotional comfort his primary concern, Dr. Leboyer developed his unique method which recognizes the moment of birth as a rite of passage. The delivery room environment for a Leboyer birth is designed to simulate the womb. It is warm, quiet and dark. Dr. Leboyer feels that although babies do not construct mental images out of what they see, they do perceive light. Being born into a brightly lit operating room is thus a shocking experience for the infant.

The most crucial difference in Dr. Leboyer's approach is that once the child is born he is placed directly on his mother's stomach with the umbilical cord still intact. The umbilicus is *not* cut until it has stopped pulsating, usually four or five minutes after birth (in standard obstetrical practices it is severed immediately). Dr. Leboyer feels that this one aspect alone makes an enormous difference for it "changes everything about the way respiration comes to the baby. If the cord is severed as soon as the baby is born, this brutally deprives the brain of oxygen. The alarm system thus alerted, the baby's entire organism reacts. Respiration is thrown into high gear as a response to aggression. Everything in the body language of the infant—in the frenzied agitation of its limbs, in the very tone of its cries—shows the immensity of its panic and its efforts to escape. Entering life, what the baby meets is death. And to escape this death it hurls itself into respiration. The act of breathing for a newborn baby is a desperate last resort. Already the first conditional reflex has been implanted, a reflex in which breathing and anguish will be associated forever." (3, p.51)

In the Leboyer method the baby, doubly supplied with oxygen (from the brain and the umbilicus), is never threatened with anoxia. Consequently, there is no panic or anguish. Not being in danger, the baby is able to relax and make a slow, gradual transition from the use of the umbilicus to the use of his lungs rather than being forced to breathe through the lungs before he is ready.

Following the cutting of the umbilical cord, the baby is placed in a 98° to 99° F. bath (similar to the temperature of the womb). The bath has a very soothing effect on the baby and soon he is able to completely relax. Once the baby is relaxed, he is dried off and dressed.

The "Birth Without Violence" approach to child delivery encourages the active participation of both parents. The father, aside from helping the mother with her breathing during the delivery, oftentimes gives the baby his first bath. This gentle, loving procedure is fast gaining acceptance in both hospital and home births.

For more information on the Leboyer method and other home birth techniques contact:

Holistic Childbirth Institute
The Holistic Life University
1627 10th Ave.
San Francisco, CA 94122
(415) 665-3200

Homebirth Inc.
89 Franklin St., Suite 200
Boston, MA 92110
(617) 482-8175

National Midwives Association
P.O. Box 163
Princeton, NJ 08540
(609) 924-1448

International Childbirth Education
    Association (ICEA)
P.O. Box 5852
Milwaukee, WI 53220

NAPSAC (National Association of Parents
    and Professionals for Safe Alternatives in
    Childbirth)
P.O. Box 1307
Chapel Hill, NC 27514
(919) 732-7302, 732-8818

Additional reading:

1. Arms, Suzanne. *Immaculate Deception.* Boston: Houghton Mifflin, 1975.
2. Gastin, Ina May. *Spiritual Midwifery.* Summertown, Tennessee: The Book Publishing Co., 1975.
3. *Leboyer, Frederick, M.D. *Birth Without Violence.* New York: Alfred A. Knopf, 1975.
4. Leboyer, Frederick, M.D. *Loving Hands—The Traditional Art of Indian Baby Massage.* New York: Alfred A. Knopf, 1976.
5. Stewart, Lee, and Stewart, David. *Safe Alternatives in Childbirth.* Chapel Hill, NC: NAPSAC Inc., 1976.
6. Stewart, Lee, and Stewart, David. *21st Century Obstetrics Now! Vol. 1.* Chapel Hill, NC: NAPSAC Inc., 1977.

Index

159

BOOKS OF RELATED INTEREST

THE HEALING MIND by Dr. Irving Oyle effectively presents an alternative to the established medical process, stating that inner belief is a vital factor in any healing process and whatever you put your faith in can be the precipitating agent for your own discovery of good health. 132 pages, soft cover, $5.95

ALPHA BRAIN WAVES by David Boxerman with Aron Spilken is a fascinating study for anyone who is interested in meditation, biofeedback or altered consciousness. It provides the reader with the current vogues and practices of the various groups using alpha brain waves. 128 pages, soft cover, $4.95

MAKING CONTACT by Virginia Satir clearly describes reliable techniques which make it possible for one to work for change in one's own perceptions, actions and life. You will learn how to understand and better use the basic tools needed to make contact with others. 96 pages, soft cover, $3.95

In **YOUR MANY FACES,** Virginia Satir demonstrates in an exciting, dramatic style how to find the key to open the door to new possibilties in our lives and how to recognize and accept the need for all our many faces — faces which reveal our inner selves. 128 pages, soft cover, $4.95

MEDICINE TODAY, HEALING TOMORROW by Dolph Ornstein, M.D. offers a visionary new concept in health care that stresses healing the patient instead of fighting the disease. He emphasizes improved nutrition, an aware sexualtiy, and the prevention of disease. 192 pages, soft cover, $4.95

Available at your local book or department store or directly from the publisher. To order by mail, send check or money order to:

Celestial Arts
231 Adrian Road
Millbrae, CA 94030

Please include $1.00 for postage and handling. California residents add 6% tax.